Copyright Kathleen Byram 2023

A Small Introduction

Hi there!

My name is Kaffy, and I'd like to be your friend.

Don't worry, just sit back and relax, because being MY friend subjects you to 24/7 LOVE.

I hope you will read this book and enjoy it thoroughly. I hope you write in the margins. That is what they are there for. If you want to draw a donkey in there, go for it. The blank spaces are for YOU, my friend.

This book can be read from start to finish, but instead, I encourage you to pick and choose what you want to read first. Just look through the table of contents and pick what looks fun to read. Nobody is saying you have to read it all, or even read it AT all. It can sit on your coffee table and remind you that you are loved. If that is all my book means to you, it's enough.

This book you hold in your hands is an instrument of love. It is meant to give you encouragement, loving feelings, ideas, and even sometimes make you angry, because life can do that.

It isn't meant to tell you from start to finish what happened to my mind and soul. Instead, take it as a series of essays, and enjoy. I believe there will be more to come.

I love you, friend, and I hope you love this book.

Dawnkey hugs

The Purpose of This Book

"It was the best of times; it was the worst of times."

That quote from Charles Dickens's *A Tale of Two Cities* describes the last few years.

Spiritually I have soared.

But there was also COVID. And death. And Trump.

I think the world has PTSD.

So, I have experienced great highs, and great lows. This is mirrored in my mental illness: having bipolar, I have experienced the same.

The purpose of this book is for you to observe these things, the highs and lows of bipolar, and the spectrum of delusion that I move up and down on. I want you to be able to observe my journey, my experiences and thoughts and feelings, and take whatever you need and want from it, and use it to your benefit.

Also, I want this book to show what is happening in the world right now. I want people to be able to read it years from now and get a good feeling for how someone felt going through it.

I also want to de-stigmatize mental illness.

Lastly, I want to share myself with my friends and family, and even the world. I have a great need, a tremendous need, to express myself and write. I would love nothing better than to share my thoughts with you.

You will come to discover that a psychotic mess can be the nicest person you'd ever hope to meet.

CONTENTS

DEDICATION

This book is dedicated to many people.

GOD.

My partner, Richard Dobscha. Without him, this wouldn't have happened.

My parents, Brenda Heath and the late Jesse Franklin Heath.

My son, of whom I am so fiercely proud, Sean Byram.

Carol Bean, my bestie and wind beneath my wings.

Nancy Price and Randi Edison, my best friends.

Ramona Smith-Kessler, my spiritual advisor and dear friend.

My beautiful family.

My Cheezfrends.

My YA friends.

My FB friends.

And everybuddy I love, which includes YOU!

Special dedication comments:

To Amy Burns, Janet Ast, Susan Himebaugh, Susan Jeswine O'Shea, Frances Young, Hector Elizalde, Ren Nawee, Christian Amatulli, John Prescott, Cindy McNash, Malcolm Hovey, Melinda Elizalde Unbehaun, Salleh Shoaf. To my dear cousin, Donna Bentley, who passed. I miss you and love you.

And lastly and very importantly, to the doctors I have loved and who have taken care of me. Drs. Jessica McCoy, Carolyn Giroux, Ryan Nicholas, and Karl Zeff, thank you for keeping me not just alive, but well and thriving. I owe so much to you all.

A Very Special Dedication to Carol Bean

Dear Carol,

This would never have happened without you. I owe so much to you. You are more than a best friend. You are everything.

You never snorted at me. You never scoffed. You never said a single negative thing.

It's been 15 years I've known you. Your love and support got me through so much. Through the suicide attempts, the self-doubt, the self-hate at times, and all of it. You were there, rain or shine. You loved me unconditionally, more than like a parent. You loved me unconditionally like The One. For

that I will be eternally grateful
and love you, you dear, dear soul.

Eternal Love,

Your Dawnkey

WHAT IS A DAWNKEY AND HOW I BECAME ONE

First, I am the only Dawnkey. There are many donkeys, but I am a DAWNKEY, and that is a special, majickal thing.

How did I come to believe such a thing about myself?

Well, I found an internet site, full of what we call LOLcat pictures, and it had lots of comments responding to each picture.

It was like a playground for me. I could write anything I wanted in those comments, and boy, did I ever.

As a rather reserved body with an ebullient soul, I felt free being able to communicate on the internet. It was the beginning of my transformation.

OK. So, I needed an avatar: some picture to represent me on the site. I thought long and hard. I wanted to be loved. That seemed to be my main goal. Who seems to be universally loved? That mouthy donkey! (You know the one).

Well, I had lots to say. Just like the talkative donkey. And boy, did I ever say it. And people liked me! And...well, it helped that I would ham it up like a donkey. People seemed to like the character! And it took on a life of its own...

I remember Mary O writing, "I love that donkey," and I felt such joy. I felt it was me that she loved.

And, in time, she did. Lots of them did. We shared love freely and liberally.

Soon it was such that people who were hurting, their hearts in need, were showing up and we were showing them a new kind of experience: a place where people on the internet are kind to you! And fun! And playful!

I think it was I who started the tradition of the Firsty Dance. People on the internet had a tendency to come along and yell "first" when they got the chance to be the first poster...it was extremely annoying. And so, it became a challenge to be first, but also say something reasonably cute or clever or whatever...not just "first." Soon a kind of thing developed where people didn't like it if you used the word First and we started jokingly saying Not Second. So, any time someone was first in the thread and didn't yell "First" we all lined up and did a dance for them! We would bring food and drinks! Have fun! Post funny things and comments! Say nice things to the poster. It became a love fest there.

I remember one special girl who didn't follow the "rules" and got first, finally, after trying and trying, and used the word "First!" and no one would dance for her.

So, I did! And I made a special point of it.

Soon afterwards she thanked me for that attention. She happened to mention in our conversation that she had been on depression medication since she was SIX. I felt so bad for her, and I was so glad I had been nice to her and treated her specially when I got that little opportunity.

It has changed back to normal since the original cheezfrends, as we called them, moved on to social media to be friends there.

The ICHC Miracle, a poem I wrote.

A poster sits before the screen

His hunger deep, his count'nance mean

His soul craves what his tongue can't ask

So fragile it must wear a mask.

Be careful what you say to him

Our new admirer

Our new cheezfrend

He sees the fun but feels alone

Greet him warmly to our home

Oh, cheezfrend, feed that hungry soul!

Bestow 5 burgers!

Fill that hole!

Encourage our friend to play and prance

When he is first, let's throw a dance!

The world is full of rude and cold

It's harsh out there!

We must be bold!

And reach out with a loving plate

Of human kindness...it's ne'er too late.

Slowwwwly...somehow, I became a Dawnkey.

DawnKey.

Now I don't know what that means to you. But it means the world to me that people would call me that.

Second, you have to remember that I am a crazy dawnkey. I tend to be a little delusional. It's a bipolar thing, I guess. And sometimes part of bipolar is feeling special. Recently, in the last couple of years, I was diagnosed with schizo-affective disorder also.

This is where the subject gets touchy, and I have trouble continuing.

See, no one wants to deal with a DONKEY that thinks it is SPECIAL. Ha! But maybe I could list WHY I think I'm special. It's not because I think I'm better than anyone. Quite the opposite, as I have learned to be very nonjudgmental. It's because I love unconditionally. I try to love every single person.

(There are some political figures that are trying my soul, but I still try to love them.) And also, to add to that love, I am effusive with praise and admiration. I love to compliment people and tell them why they matter, and that they DO matter. My God, how you matter, my friend. Never forget that the teensiest little action that you perform could cause ripples that will manifest a miracle.

Which brings me to...

Ripples

Have you ever been so blessed to have the experience of doing something and then seeing the ever-widening results, like ripples in the water? A tiny stone thrown into the stagnant water causes a ripple effect.

Our daily deeds are like that. The tiniest little actions, that we never stop to give a thought to, have great ripple effects we will never know. The ripples go out and touch others, causing them to touch others, and on and on it goes.

My first true and significant realization of how my actions really affect others, and how, as my mother would tell me, "People are always watching," was when I married my first husband at eighteen. I was painfully ignorant and immature. I lived in a very small town (2,000) and everyone knew everyone else's business. I received a card in the mail. It said, "The merchants of Orleans have contributed to a Family Bible for you as a wedding gift." Now, I was not particularly religious at that point in my life, or even that spiritual. I was an ostrich. But I was deeply touched at this lovely gesture, and I filled out the card and mailed it in.

I received a beautiful white Bible with our name in it. I was not about to read it, haha! But I appreciated the love, intention, concern, and other motivations behind it. I felt gratitude.

My mother had instilled in me the necessity of writing thank-you notes.

I wrote thank-you letters to every single merchant that contributed to that Bible.

Now, as you can imagine, that town had a depressed economy. It was tough to find a job. Our best market was run by a real go-getter who only employed the most winning personalities—kids from my high school—the ones that made everyone smile. I was a reserved, quiet child. I did not exude that charm. But I had put in my application anyway, and of course, was not called.

Soon after that thank you letter went out, I was hired.

Just think about that. That simple little Thank You note. Now think about this: how many people do you think sent them a thank-you note for their Bible?

This really does not fit in with my subject today, but it feels like an important prelude. It made me aware of how my simple actions could touch others. Here are some more things I have picked up over time that I am aching to share with you, about kindness and affecting others, which is at the cornerstone of my DawnKeyness.

In my senior yearbook, a girl I barely noticed from my art class wrote, "To the most considerate person I ever met." I cried, and never forgot it. Later I realized her last name was that of the family who was friends with my mother's side of the family.

When I moved from Indianapolis, from a huge school with some cruel children, to Orleans, a tiny school (my class had only 50), I noticed a stunning difference in the personalities of the children. They were not hateful to each other. They did not mock. They had decent upbringings and mores.

I made friends with a neighbor girl and her friend, who rode the bus with me but were still in the lower school, a few grades behind. I gave them nicknames. "Sarah Hare" and "Joy

Robin"…(as you can see, I have not outgrown my connection with the significance of avatars…). One day on the bus they passed me a note. I had not received many notes as a child, being reserved, a little odd, and not given to being cheerful or very outwardly friendly, so I was titillated with happiness! I rushed into the house and opened it. It was, really, my friends, a love letter. It was covered with stickers and said, "We like our names you gave us!" and "We're glad you're our friend!" and other things. I had never in my life received anything like that. I sat and cried.

I was a home health aide in southern Indiana years later. One man, Mr. L, loved his aides and was grateful for them. His words belied this, but his body and expressions did not. His body and affect were stiff. I do not know his diagnosis. He was like a stone. I knew much was going inside that prison of a body he was trapped in....

One day he expressed his angst at his predicament. He wondered what use he was. Why was he even alive? Useless, useless...he thought. My heart almost broke for him. Oh, Mr. L! I told him, with great emotion. I am sure my whole, normally reserved, manner exploded with expression. You have no idea what plans are made for you! You have no idea what effect your tiny little actions might have upon the world! One tiny little thing that you think nothing of may cause a ripple effect that will spread out and cause a major effect that will change the world!!

His stiff, stone-like body collapsed inwards, in a heap, and he *howled*! "HUUUUUNNNNNNHHHHH!"

I shook with the knowledge of what I had affected in his spirit. I will never forget, in a million years.

Other beautiful things:

When I was eight months pregnant in August in Indianapolis, living in hell, my then husband had some trouble and was separated from me. I was alone. No air conditioning. No stove. No food. No hot water. No brain. We were insane with stress.

The next-door neighbor of our duplex came and knocked on the door. He lived with his children and their mother. He was a nice man. He took me to his home. He led me upstairs to their air-conditioned bedroom and told me to take a nap. When I awoke, he served me dinner in bed. Not long after, my mom and cousin came up with the station wagon and moved me out of there and took me back home to Orleans.

Bob on Tacoma in Indianapolis in 1989, God Bless your soul. I hope you are happy wherever you are.

In San Francisco I managed a bakery (now closed) in Pacific

Heights. A customer began to come, who acted strangely. I thought perhaps what he suffered from was something like Tourette's. I had the funniest intuition/imagination that when others came around, he would worry that he would have a "spell," and the nervousness would bring it on. I would save my coffee bean grinding for his visits. I would keep a peripheral eye on him, and when it seemed right, would turn on the loud grinding machine, and no one could hear any odd sounds, and no one could be embarrassed for making them. I do not know if he knew I was trying to work with him. I hope he did and that that was why he kept coming back. For a while. Then I suspect the owner, not much of a Donkey type, spied him one day and it was all she wrote.

I remember a lovely lady, a co-worker of sorts, that sadly left for Arizona. I guess I was not aware of the level of my affection for her. One day when calling her from one store to 'clear' before coming, she answered and I blurted out with uncharacteristic verbal enthusiasm, "Hello my sweet friend!"

Dead silence. My face burned and eyes popped with horror at my schmucky, cringey, dorky act and self.

When I got to the store, there was a piece of paper in my parts box. It had a childlike drawing of a smiley face—highlighters had been used to enhance it. My eyes began to sting a little. I said without thinking, "Who did this?" and a co-worker said, "I think she did."

She was sitting in front of the computer. She would not look at me. We were stiff with our embarrassment at the emotion of the situation.

I told her, "I have a special place for things like this, that I put special things in. I will keep this." And she nodded, smiling.

Isn't it funny, the little things that happen that touch you so deeply? And that you remember?

The quality of your life can explode with intensity when you begin living to love. Just little acts can have such an impression, and you never know who is watching or being affected, and how they will go on and touch someone else.

I share these things that touch me so that I may touch you and that they will make a difference.

Live your life as though the people who matter to you are watching.

And now, maybe you understand a little more about Dawnkiness, but I suspect I still wasn't very clear.

OK, I'll start back at the beginning.

Uh oh, going to have to digress. Where is the beginning? Well, I suspect that it happened infinity or so years ago, from our Maker. I like to think sparks of our Maker, called spirits, come to earth and humanify our bodies, breathing life into a soul.

Or something. Your experience may vary.

At any rate, I've been around, and I suspect, so have you. Many, many times. So that we can learn things and experience things we cannot in heaven.

Earth seems to be a tradeoff. Icky stuff can happen, but the highs are just...*magnificent*.

So, yes, the beginning.

I was born 6/25/65 in Frankfurt, Germany.

My mother had wanted me since she was 16 years old. She badly wanted a girl. When she married dad, at 23 or 24, and they were shipped out to Germany, she went on the birth control pill. Her doctor gave it to her because she explained she did not want to get pregnant and be throwing up while traveling, and this made sense to him. So, she went on the pill.

Well, I was up in heaven waiting. I knew she would be my mother. I know I must have been so excited to go because she is such a stellar mother.

Mom said the night she conceived me a light came down, warming her, and she knew that I was inside her. She knew she was pregnant, even though she was on the pill.

She bled. She went to the doctor, terrified that she was losing me. Oh, puh! Like I had any intention of leaving! I had business to attend to!

She was sooo careful with me. I bet she didn't even have coffee.

She would have nightmares. At some point she thought there was a lion under her bed. This was shocking because she's always been so...pragmatic? Sane? Level-headed! That's definitely her...

I was born in June. I was due on the 9th. I did not come until the 25th, and that was only because dad wanted to know if he could lift her if he needed to. He picked her up and her water broke, and she went to the hospital where I was born. No telling how long I'd have stayed if that hadn't happened. I was delivered with forceps. I like to imagine that I didn't want to come out of there.

I was a sensitive child.

When dad would scream and yell, mom said I would hold my breath and pass out. The doctor said to let me do it.

Have you ever tried to do that? When you were in severe pain and wanted to pass out? It doesn't work.

Yeah, I'm still pouting about it.

I bet I was my mom's best friend. She was almost always mine. Actually, I have several best friends. I have my bestest best friend, Carol Bean, and my best friends Randi and Nancy, and it's like a trinity. I've had best friends before. But my mom was my first best friend in this life and will be 'til the end.

She was very alone.

This is a woman who was the oldest out of ten children. She is also bossy. How could she not be? But this woman, this woman is Queen of Bossy! I've never seen such a great delegator.

But she didn't learn everything overnight. She had a process. Like me.

She is the best, most magnificent mother in the world.

Get used to hyperbole from me. You will find it often.

Anyway, back to Germany. She was stuck in that little apartment with me and had nothing to do but clean house and play with me.

She was HAPPY. She loved me so much.

Things were hard, too.

As I mentioned the screaming before, Dad wasn't perfect. Mom was perfect, okay? But not dad. Dad was human. And dad was fussy. She tells of how she would fix a nice hot breakfast for him and repeatedly try to get him to get up to eat it, until it would turn cold, and he'd hop out of bed, go to the table, and complain that it was too cold and said he couldn't eat it. She couldn't fix him more because she had to leave.

He would go through the apartment with a white glove. He would move things. Just a hair. She would put something somewhere. Maybe she did it to cover a spot or something. I'm making that up for an example. A spot probably didn't dare show its face in her clean apartment. Anyway, he had a little weird thing that he would adjust things "just so." He was fastidious. He was a Felix Unger.

She remembers working one day hand sewing a precious pair of curtains from some fabric she had and put them up over an ugly window. He came home and tore them down and called them…something hideous and ugly. She was mortified.

He would call her stupid. Mom is not stupid. Because she was so loving to me throughout my life, I never noticed just how smart she was until I got much, much older.

Waits while you older folks laugh knowingly

So finally, mom said to him, "You're a smart man. Why would you want a stupid wife?" and he never said it again.

She adored me. She was so happy to have me. The only thing I remember from this time is sitting in the kitchen sink, playing with the water.

My next memory is in Atlanta, I think...I was about 4? And trying on my dad's Xray pants. I remember thinking about how long before they would fit.

Atlanta wasn't a happy place for mom. Grandma (dad's mom) tried to control her. Dad couldn't be himself around her. Things got bad and they moved. I know we lived in Virginia and Indianapolis.

And that brings me to...

FITTING IN

The term "fitting in" brought to mind two different scenarios. First, I thought of high school and how I believed I was perceived. The second, I thought of literally "fitting in" to a chair. I'll leave that for a small separate paper, which I hope will be met with good-natured humor.

So, onto high school we go.

The story begins in 1979. That was a funky year. It was the ending of disco and the 70s, and the beginning of the torrid 80s. I remember a friend singing, "Disco, disco sucks ♪" in class that fall of '79. He was wearing corduroys probably, and the flannel plaid shirt, most likely.

I'd like to give you a small social, culturally eye-opening description of that time, but that's not what this is about. This is about me and how I "fit in."

Well, I didn't.

At least that was how it felt. It always kinda felt that way.

My first day of high school I looked awesome. I looked like Annie Hall or something. But not that funky. More conservative. I especially remember the shoes. They looked like a banker's shoes...wingtips? My pants were pleated, a soft material, tweedy. Very dressy yet casual. And a mauve blouse with a Henley neckline. Unfortunately, I was still burdened with glasses, but at least they weren't a million years old.

I looked so snazztastic that as I walked up the steps of my school one of my middle school mates turned and did a double take. That made me feel fantastic. Well, I still remember it, some 40 years later.

I had friends that year. Several girls who I joined at lunch time to eat with and talk with. We weren't the most popular girls, but we were nice girls. We were normal girls. We were the girls guys secretly asked out because they were comfortable and friendly.

Except I was also prickly and odd.

I was delighted when flirted with.
I was 14. I never held somebody's
hand romantically, never been
romantically kissed.

(When I was probably around 8
or 9 my friend and I decided to
touch tongues. This was the most
bold and outrageous thing we
could think of to do. So! We did
it! And then promptly fell about
the place in paroxysms of spasms
and protests at the ickiness. We
might have done this more than
once.)

I was a fun kid. I think I fit in well
as a child, before I got odd
around middle school. LOL.

I was fun in the neighborhood. I
was also trustworthy. I was
quickly passed around as a

reliable and fun babysitter that children liked.

It was because I related to children as a child. I always relate to others as a child.

[1]Eric somebody had this model of how people communicate. There were parents, children, and adults. It showed different ways that people communicate. For example, I usually present as a child to another child. Or as a child to a parent. They in turn, may choose to respond as a child, as in, "Hey yeah, let's do it!" OR they might respond like a parent, chiding me. Or an adult, maturely and logically.

---

[1] Editor's note: Eric Berne's PAC (parent-adult-child) model of communication.

I NEVER relate to people as a parent. I don't have that vibe in me. More on that another time.

Usually, I was childlike with a reserved, adult-like manner. I'm telling you; I was odd. LOL.

I liked the normal things children liked, growing up. I did make up games. I enjoyed doing that. I made up fun board games too. I remember sliding down the carpeted steps on a cardboard, maybe? And my friend hurt her tailbone. I remember making up The Ghost of Hamlet game (don't ask how I came up with that as an 8- or 9-year-old) where I would get under a blanket and the kids would come up and tease me and poke at me and sometimes, I would rear up suddenly, making them scream and laugh and run, and it was great fun.

I suddenly remembered that my mother was a day care mother. She had a little day care in their own home.

So, I was older than the other kids. I felt like the Big Cheese.

I remember when I was in the Brownies (like Girl Scouts?) and was on the Debbie Show. Mom's day care kids got to watch me on there. It must have been very cool for them to see me on tv.

I had an 8-Ball. You know, the one with the blue or green creepy fluid inside and the pyramid says your answer on it.

I loved that 8-Ball.

I also loved bouncing. There was a boy in our complex when I was in first grade, and he had a rubber bouncy ball with a handle on it. I was CRAZY for that bouncy ball. I wanted to bounce it soooo bad. I'd never been on a trampoline or a pogo stick, at that age, yet. I just always had this desire, this neeeeed, to BOUNCE! Like a Tigger!!

So, I politely asked him if I could bounce on his ball.

Nope.

This was news. Okay, regroup.

What if...What if...what if that? Or this?

Nope, nope, nopety nope.

Yes, I suspect now that he was a little buttface.

This gets worse.

I finally was so desperate to bounce on that ball, that I offered him my beloved 8 ball in return for a BOUNCE. ONE BOUNCE. And finally, he grudgingly accepted. It was a cruel tease of a victory.

Later, as I was donking about as was my wont, I happened upon one of those holes in the bottom of the building, with the metal around it. I don't know how to explain it. Anyway, I looked down.

There was my beloved 8-Ball, broken, at the bottom.

That broke my heart. And somehow, it felt wrong, like *I* was the one who had messed up here. I had a lovely thing and threw it away for a fling. I felt like I betrayed my 8-Ball friend. That's how it felt.

I had a tendency always to anthropomorphize things. I didn't care much for dolls, but I loved stuffed animals. I couldn't lay anything that looked like a living being on the floor askew, its face down. I had to lay them carefully, always.

Anyway, back to fitting in.

I must have gotten another 8-Ball (yay!) because one year we spray painted it silver and I played a fortune teller at our friend's carnival. I think she did it to raise money for [2]MD. I think. Anyway, that was very exciting for me, getting dressed up with makeup and all and playing this fortune teller.

Later, in our yard one day, I set up a table and a sign saying I would tell someone's fortune for 50 cents, or something like that. A very jolly, large man came by in his big car.

He reminded me of a friend of ours, so maybe that's why I liked him.

He was very good-natured. He howled when I looked at his palm and said he would have XX

---

[2] Muscular Dystrophy

number of children. He enjoyed himself thoroughly.

I always remembered that kind, jolly fellow.

I was a fun kid. But my friends were growing up. I wasn't.

I remember standing out in the dark with my friends on the street when we were pre-teens. There was a boy in our group who I liked, but my friend got him instead. I didn't resent her for this one tiny bit. I don't know how that could be...interesting. Anyway, that night we were hanging about, being us, and I suddenly thought of a joke. I whispered to my friend to tell her guy, "You need a new butt. Your old one has a crack in it."

This was incredibly hilarious to me. I thought they would love it, too.

She told him.

He took his foot and violently shoved his skateboard INTO HER SHIN.

She did not flinch. Did not say a word. Just looked at him.

I did not understand the psychology behind all this, or the sexuality, or anything. I was just hurt as hell at what he had done, and later grateful I had not been his girl.

Anyway, that sums up how I felt. Like an outsider who didn't understand things.

BUT!

When I was around 11, I went to the mall with my friend. (At this point I still had several friends, but always had one special friend. Pisces people seemed particularly vibey with me.) We went to the bookstore, and I found [3]*Everything You Always Wanted to Know About Sex* (* But Were Afraid to Ask)*. Oh, yes. I found it. And I was clinically interested.

Not horny. Not trying to score. Just feeling that it was time I understood all this. Sneaking my mom's COSMO magazines and my dad's Playboys wasn't doing the trick.

------

3 David R. Reuben M.D., 1969

(Yes, I believe he sincerely kept those for the fiction.)

Anyway! I was at the bookstore, no older than 12, probably 11, and I talked the clerk into letting me buy it!!!!!

How did I manage this? I very calmly and rationally explained to her that my mother would approve because she was very open-minded and would want me learning from a doctor, who wrote the book. She sold it to me!

I couldn't just read it and keep my mouth shut. I always told my mom EVERY thing.

So, I told her about it, and she took it away and gave it to Aunt Martha. Never saw it again.

I'm digressing.

I think I had my share of being liked when I was young. I don't know about when I got older.

Around 11 or 12, sixth grade middle school, I started feeling VERY uncomfortable. Girls looked hot and they were attracting boys. I did not look hot. For one thing, except for getting out of the house once in purple velvet pants and purple suede boots, I did not dress popularly.

I dressed weird.

One time I wore purple polyester KNIT pants, with a purple and blue madras shirt, which I loved, and had to wear my brown rubber boots because it was raining.

I forgot my shoes.

I had to wear brown rubber boots with polyester knit pants all day. That's the schmucky way I was.

When I was in eighth grade, I started to get more comfortable again.

Until ninth.

Then, in 1979, I saw a guy in my class that I was insane for.

I started dressing like I thought he would dress.

Elsewhere I mention about my dad–that I would try to identify with him, a male, instead of my mom, a female. I did the same with this guy.

Instead of wanting to look nice, I wanted to look like him.

I was wildly infatuated with him.
He would torment me. It was
awful, and I think I was highly
impressionable, and it molded
me in a twisted way.

Enough of that.

Moving on to Orleans, Indiana, in
1980.

It was a culture shock.

For one thing, it was un-
airconditioned. I got sent home
(to Aunt Jenny's across the
street) every time I'd get swollen
up from hives from being hot. Or
got a migraine.

And yet these kids did not treat
me like a weirdo.

They were so nice. The first that
was so kind to me was TB. I had

friends. People who liked me. I didn't have to go to PE and show them how uncoordinated I was.

I never felt comfy in my own body.

And I abused it horribly. But that's for another story.

Around third grade, I think, was when dad got health-kicky, and our diets changed.

That was when I got yearny for food, and the weight started to grow. I was always a little plump. When I was 15, I was about a 14/16. They didn't have cool clothes for heavier people then. Still, I was never made fun of for my clothes.

This was a poor area. Meaning monetarily. A southern Indiana farming area.

I thought I was prettier than I was. And sometimes slathered on the makeup. I hated my glasses. I felt like such a goob.

Senior year I was able to show up in contacts. I was so happy with myself I could burst. I finally felt like I could show everybody my beautiful face.

I was vain.

I remember saying to my best friend at the time that I was finally pretty. She gave me a look, and I quickly said, "You know what I mean," and was ashamed.

My vanity was very insecure.

I've always been insecure.

It's what drives my feeling
alienated from my friends, when
they were always right there
loving me the whole time.

Snippets of Life

I remember Mrs. Morgan.

I was sitting cross-legged on the floor with the other children. It was third grade (or fourth? hmm). It was English class. I was always great in English. I had our book out in front of me, and it was fascinating, and I was thumbing through it. I must have been bored, listening to a child trying to read or something like that. Out of the sky like a thunderbolt I felt a hand grabbing my arm and snatching me up, pulling me up off the floor, and dragging me across the room to another room where she shut the door and gave me hell.

When finished, she asked, not kindly, if I wanted to stay in there a bit. I said no and followed her back. Everyone was looking at me. Twerphead McGee (an alias), my nemesis, said with excitement, "I think she's going to cry!" and that is all I remember of that.

Twerphead McGee, his new name, was a little, you guessed it! twerp head, and tried to make my life miserable.

One day my friend and I chased around a boy whose name escapes me now, trying to catch him so she could kiss him. I was puzzled as to why he was not interested in being kissed by my friend. He loudly called out that he was being chased, in fakey sort of voice about it, and I thought he was protesting too much. I do not remember how this went.

The next day, it seems, I was at the swings and some children surrounded me. Twerphead McGee was there. I called him a punk. Several children closed in on me, all calling me punk. I lay on the swing to swing back and forth, and J. sat on my back. They howled with laughter. That is all I remember that day.

The next day, I told some friends what happened, and they were angry.

At recess, the crowd came up. My crowd stepped up, too. There was a tussle. I remember two girls, fingers locked over each other's hands, struggling with each other.

This, too, I don't remember the rest of…

It took me a long time to put two and two together and figure out they were trying to avenge their friend who we playfully chased for a kiss.

T. McGee was definitely a pill.

One of my parents told me to wait until he was just about to do something bad to me, then yell out his name.

So, the next day, we were standing in line, boys and girls, I think. He was across from me. It was winter, and we were dressed for it.

T took his black leather glove and slowly removed one finger at a time, as he calmly prepared to slap me with it across the space between us. I watched with interest as he planned his heinous little act. I waited, like a spider. Juuuust as he pulled back and was about to strike, I yelled out his name, TWERPHEAD MCGEE! And the teacher whirled around! And she caught him, mid-slap! Muahahahah!! He was taken to the front of the line. I do not know what happened to him.

It was in fifth grade that I stopped getting my nose rubbed in the carpet when I had to clean my room.

This was because my father found out I needed glasses. I was failing math. I couldn't see the board.

Something strange happened regarding that starting in third grade.

We had a teacher, Mrs. C, who went through a divorce and ended up leaving. She must have been my math teacher, because soon Mrs. J became our teacher. Oddly, all I remember of her was her reading us stories. I don't remember learning anything that year. In fourth grade, I was lost. Couldn't do the work. I felt like I missed something. In fifth grade, I failed math.

So, I got glasses, and all of a sudden, I could see the board. And my grade started raising. By eighth grade I had an A.

I don't remember a lot from fifth grade. A few instances, things not worth sharing. Sixth grade was another story.

I was funky cringey awkward. In my sixth-grade pic I had a fro, ugly silver framed glasses, and a brown polyester knit dress with a huge lace collar, and the dress came up mid-thigh. I looked a FOOL.

Once, I wore some purple velvet pants I got a hold of, with some purple suede boots the neighbor lady gave us.

Some kid asked my friend if I was a stripper.

Another time, my lost-friend B and her new friend watched as I approached their lunch table toward the lunch line. They stopped me and asked if I was a virgin. I was wearing forest green polyester gabardine pants, with a little frog sewn on a hole I had gotten in my pants. Sixth grade. A virgin? I stopped, stunned. My mind freaked. A virgin? What's a virgin? I was stupefied for a minute. They laughed uproariously. "She has to think about it!!"

Sixth grade was hard.

I almost forgot about M. He was annoying, that one. He constantly threatened to knock my glasses off. He would keep saying, "Hit me. Hit me." And I would just get angry. One day, some people were around, and he said it, so I did. I hit him. And he promptly smacked at my glasses. The fight was about to ensue, and our friends pulled us apart. I am sure it was a hilarious scene.

I had a bully, of course, as many of us probably did. This bully I will call Little Twerp. LT liked to punch me in the arm for silly offenses and threaten me and walk in front of me.

One time she and a friend stood at my locker on both sides of me, punching me in the arms. All of a sudden, I had a nervous breakdown.

I howled.

I was vaguely aware of the kerfluffle it caused. One girl ran and got a teacher. Don't remember a lot after that, but LT got talked to.

I talked to my dad about LT. He informed me that I needed to kick her butt down the hall next time she walked in front of me like that again.

So one day B's new friend was chatting me up at a table at breaktime, and I decided to talk to her about LT. I informed her that the next time Little T came up and started sloooowly walking in front of me, I was going to take the ball of my foot, apply it to her ass, and propel her in an arc up into the air and down the hall. Very clinically and drolly I informed her of this. It was quite impressive sounding.

I never got bullied again.

Except at the end of school, she came to me and said, "I'm gonna get _____" (a girl we both knew) and showed me a knife in her locker. I thought, "Oh, no you aren't," and informed the office. The next year she was gone.

In seventh grade I got my first pair of jeans. They were hideous and I looked like a foo. They did nothing for my shape. I lusted for Levis. Straight legged Levis. Too expensive. Sigh. So I looked like a lumpy dump.

In eighth grade I started to come out of my shell, just a teensy teensy bit. I actually went to a school dance and thought about dancing at one point.

In ninth grade, I was struck by a huge crush.

I walked into math class and the most attractive guy I'd seen was sitting there. Instead of my normal routine, I walked right up and sat behind him.

Soon he and his friends were harassing me and calling me a slut and a whore and throwing things at me in class.

This was hard and confusing for me. I was a virgin, I was very reserved, I had never even held a guy's hand, and I was stunned. It was particularly bad because I was attracted to him. I believe this experience did something weird to me.

That year, I believe, my friend N's mother died. That was horrible. Then we moved away from her, leaving her behind. It was awful.

She came and lived with us down in southern Indiana.

It was very exciting at first. But my friend's mother had died, and she was in crisis. I did not have enough sense to know how to deal with it, and I dealt with it poorly. Really poorly.

We had an attic room. It was very cozy.

School in southern Indiana was different from Indianapolis. Next, I'll tell you about that.

My first day of school.

OK, I'm from Indianapolis. I'm used to going to an air-conditioned school, and in September.

We were in southern Indiana. It's a little warmer down there.

There was no AC.

OMG. I was a perfect little snowflake.

I had red corduroy pants on. They were really pretty. They were also hot. I was also wearing a red multi-colored plaid blouse with a button-up lacy collar. I was not comfortable. I was hot, and red was a little bold for me, but I wanted to look nice for my new classmates.

I remember walking through the hall and some jerky kid passed me in the busy hall. He said something like, you're trying to show off by wearing red pants.

Another boy I didn't know, but knew of, asked me if I partied. I did not know at the time that that meant doing drugs. I said I didn't have time. I wasn't attracted to him and thought that he was testing the waters for a date, which I wasn't interested in, but I didn't want to be rude.

Then there was S. Oh, God, was he ever there. He looked like a scarecrow. He had straw-like hair, and his face was scarred everywhere, and he was too thin and angular.

He did strange things.

He would take his finger and stick it in your face (in the outside corner of your eye) and shake. He would "throw" spit at people. He was hyper and strange.

I wanted to kill him. I did not love everyone back then like I do now.

He had a girl give me a note he had written.

He said he liked my "bobblers," and was sorry for giving me a "hard time," and when he got his car would I go with him?

I said nothing. I was appalled. I was especially appalled that my very first love letter was from 1. S, and 2. talked about "bobblers."

Once, in ninth grade (the year before), I received a triangular note from a boy I found attractive in my class. I was THRILLED. Before I could open it, there was the teacher, demanding it. I never got to find out what was in that letter. I still resent that teacher for doing that. My self-esteem would have soared if I could have read something.

One other letter came from a friend of S. I was not attracted, nor interested in his mind, as I didn't know anything about him, except that he was friends with S. This did not help his cause, as I was suspicious of a guy that would screw his friend over that way, asking the girl he liked out.

Years later I was working in Subway in French Lick, and I was taking a smoke break out back. There was another employee there.

Suddenly, strangers, a man and a woman, were standing out there with me, wanting to be waited on. The employee had gone to the bathroom and not warned me, and these customers got tired of waiting and came looking for someone.

Guess whose parents they were.

S would have laughed his freaking guts out if he had seen this happen.

S did laugh his freaking guts out once...our classmate A, an amiable sort, was the victim of a perm. He had jet straight hair. It looked like someone bent it. It was hilarious.

S died young and it was sad. I wish I could have known him on a friendlier level and not been aggravated with him. I think he was probably a very sarcastic, funny person.

My first friends at OHS were on the bus. They were younger than I, and may have been in elementary school, but one was a neighbor. She was so friendly and fun. I loved them both. I used to enjoy going down to her house to visit.

One day, when I was new to the school, a girl asked me what my friends called me. I snobbily responded, "My NAME is Kathleen." To which she said, aside to her friends, "That's a snob," which, of course, she was right. My friend stood up for me though! She fiercely said good things about me. I was so touched.

It felt like everyone was family, close or extended. And some of them were.

One boy, who seemed popular and was kind of cute, was sitting behind me. He took a film strip from the projector or something and looped it around my neck from behind.

I turned around and gave him the slow Nic Cage head turn. I stared at him. I think he blushed. This was all I did. I heard in my ear another nice-looking boy call out softly in a friendly tone, "He's flirting with you ♪" and I only kind of half-registered it, psyche-wise. This was hard to accept. And I was so uncomfortable in my body. I felt so strange.

Some people were richer than others, some better looking, some smarter, so on and so forth, but there wasn't a clique in our class that I knew of. We had nice people in our class.

One time, though, something troubling happened.

I was in a "mixed" class of grades. I remember an older boy was in there, sitting behind me, and another boy in my grade sitting in front of me. The boy behind me, J#1, had a piece of molding. He was poking J#2, in front of me. It was getting in my way, too, and annoying me besides.

Now, I wouldn't have gotten involved, except that I had a massive love for J#2. J#1 could go hang. But J2 was good quality stuff.

So, at the end of class, when the bell rang, J2 jumped up and proceeded to attempt to kick J1's butt.

I don't know who came out worse. All I know is I was brought to the principal's office and grilled. I informed them of the truth.

I paid for that dearly.

One day, in that class, S was harassing me and throwing things at me, making my skin prickle and my heart race with fear, and a girl tapped my shoulder and said, "There's a bunch of girls after you." To which I burst out laughing.

I thought she meant S could have gotten any girl he wanted.

What she meant was that girls wanted to beat me up, because J1 was handsome and popular and a star athlete.

We were allowed knives in that country type school.

So, I carried a big one.

But I think what kept me from getting beaten up was The English Assignment.

The English Assignment was to take a box and make it about you. And so, I did.

And I got up in front of the class and made a fool of myself. OK, that's what it felt like. And I think they saw that I was human.

I honestly believe that saved me.

I really didn't want to have to use that knife.

I made a friend whose name was Susan. She lived in town. We had fun. She had a fun adult boyfriend, and he had a friend named T. T was scruffy.

Yes, scruffy is the best word right now.

The first time I met him, my very first date, I was 17. I was shown a picture of a pleasant looking guy with a sideways-broken nose in a camel-colored suit, if I recall it correctly.

I said okay.

So, I met him by stepping into Susan's boyfriend's car and he was sitting there.

He looked a mess.

Later he said he did it so I would accept him as he was, sort of. I could understand that.

I was not pleased when he kissed me. It was my first, and it was icky.

I ended up marrying him.

I ended up divorcing him not long after.

I was horrible. Horrible.

Yes, I truly was.

I would get my bank statement in the mail and throw it in the desk. I didn't have the brains to do the statement. I just didn't think about it.

I did lots of bad stuff. I was immature and selfish and just...bad.

It is good for him that I divorced him.

I married him at 18, divorced by 21.

At the age of 21 I began to show strange signs of mental illness.

Advice From a Dawnkey

I am loath to give advice.

But a little ego steps in and says, "Dawnkey, you might have some good points to make."

And then my cowardly little cynic inside says, "But you'll make people mad if you try to tell them what to do."

See, that's why I show my process. I tell you what I experienced, and you, in turn, take what you need, leave what you don't.

So instead of saying, "Do this" I am actually saying, "*I* did this, and you can use that information for your own gain, if you so choose."

Here are some random things I'd like to share with you:

1. I have found listening to be priceless. I learned to listen, as my father always tried to impress on me.

2. I learned to carefully pick my battles. So many things aren't worth squat compared to losing a friend.

3. I have learned that being kind to mean people can bring beautiful results.

4. Some people are bound and determined to be mean no matter what you do/say. I have learned that not engaging in verbal combat reduces the problems.

5. About 15 years ago someone told me that Love is a Choice. I immediately rejected that. Then I accepted it. Then I adopted it, and found it got easier and easier to love people. Now I either love or try to love everybuddy as much as I can.

6. I don't know if everything happens for a reason, but I know that so much can be learned from bad things that happen, even when it happens to good people. Sometimes we don't even know we learned something, until it's time for that skill set to make itself needed and you reach down inside you and find tools you didn't

know were there! And you succeed! Or maybe your bad experience makes the next time easier. And it gets easier and easier. I find myself looking constantly for meaning and purpose.

7. It does something to the psyche to be told repeatedly (several times a day) "I love you!" in a loving and/or positive way.

8. People's names are important to them. I make an effort to say and spell people's names correctly.

9. Art is a wonderful expression. You don't have to be good at it to do it. There is no reason why you can't just throw a bunch of colors you

like on a canvas and frame it
and hang it and be proud of
how you captured your
feeling/thoughts and
managed to convey it to your
audience. I have a house full
of my paintings, and they
aren't professional grade.
Heck, I can't even make
clouds. But I love being
surrounded by my paintings.
I highly recommend painting
or finding artistic endeavors
to pursue. It's a great way of
expressing yourself and
keeping track of it and your
progression.

10. I apologize when I'm
wrong. Maybe I apologize too
much. But it doesn't seem to
be doing any harm...

11. Oh, geez, I almost forgot. Compliment people. Make it genuine. (Don't lie about it. People can see through you, even if they don't consciously recognize it sometimes, they do subconsciously, and it drives their motivation.)

12. Oh, yeah. I have a real problem if I have to lie. It is unbelievably hard for me to do. This seems to serve me well. I don't consider all omissions to be lies, either. If someone says, "What do you think of my hair?" and I don't care for it, but I think it's interesting, that's what I'll say: that I think it is interesting. I won't throw in the part that I don't care for

it. What would be the purpose of that? I won't lie and say, "OMG I LOVE YOUR HAIR!" I just don't do that. It's not genuine and that's not Dawnkish.

Dawnkish= be honest until it's going to hurt, and then keep your mouth shut unless it's necessary to say. Basically, if you can't say anything good, don't say anything? Well, sometimes bad things need to be said. I'm not usually a 100% gung-ho type of person about statements. I see exceptions and sometimes people fall in the exception area and need to feel valid and recognized.

13. Face your fear! (OK, I got bossy on that one.) This is what I recommend you try. Sometimes people have luck with doing it in increments. Others need to jump straight in. Still others are helped by talking about it. There are all kinds of ways to try facing your fear. Your effort is what means the most. What if you fail? No worries: you made next time easier by your effort.

14. I tend not to speak in absolutes.

15. Creative Visualization for things that are hurting you. I have a very vivid and active imagination. (BTW I don't know if it

gets stronger by exercising it, but it doesn't hurt to try!) What Creative Visualization means to ME is basically fantasizing at a high emotional pitch. Using vivid fantasy as a healing balm for your heart. I'll discuss this subject more at length later.

16.Ask not for whom the bell tolls, it tolls for thee. Or as someone else said, "There ARE no others." What does this mean to me? We are all one.

SPORTS

I dislike sports.

Now, before anybuddy gets their feelers hurt, I'd like to say I kind of admire sports in a way. Because it is the glue that holds some families together. It can also get a poor kid a scholarship. And it's good for you. Lots of things. Teamwork (not good at that) and camaraderie.

That said:

When I was around 2 or 3 or so, my mother watched me jump off a high dive. She said she almost had a nervous breakdown. She had put me in swimming lessons. I took to water very well. You could say I've a bit of an obsession with it sometimes.

It was in elementary gym, however, that I discovered I did not have the Sports Bug, or whatever you want to call it. First, those gym suits. OH GOD DID I HATE THOSE. I was not built for gym suits. And I looked like a little blob whilst everyone around was svelte. Hmph.

Oh, I tried basketball, around fifth grade or so maybe? I was in C group. I'll let you figure out what THAT means. I liked it. Basketball was fun. But I wasn't very adept. I was kinda clumsy. I remember people yelling, "Heath!" at me in anger and disgust, annoyance and impatience. I was the type that tries to push when it says PULL.

Mom decided I needed dance lessons. I took tap, jazz, and ballet. I liked it. I enjoyed getting up and performing in front of people, but especially I liked the fancy suits! Later I was so sick with nerves mom stayed up with me all night.

I liked field hockey and soccer. I did not like the dark red rubber dodge balls. The bigger boys threw them HARD. I was terrified of one smashing my bespectacled face.

In ninth grade I took a full year of P.E. When I moved from that school to Orleans High School, in Orleans, Indiana, there was quite a kerfluffle of confusion on what to do with me, because kids only took PE part time and Health part time. So, I got to go to Health and to Study Hall instead of P.E.

And that's when I became more confident. I could hide my (I thought gross) body and nobody could see it in the locker room. No one could yell at me in the gym or on the field because I was being a doofus.

I was just never that athletic. I liked gymnastics. That appealed to me. And I loved using the trampoline and doing flips.

I remember the Crab Ball in elementary school. I LOVED that Crab Ball. We would get on the floor and walk like crabs and kick the ball around and it would bounce us: it was a huge tarp or canvas, maybe, covered ball. Did you guys ever have a crab ball?

And climbing the rope. I really enjoyed that and was good at it.

Running around the track? Nope nope nope. I was always last.

I was a bookish and creekish kid. I liked to read on my bed, I liked stuffed animals, I liked art, and I liked going down to the creek.

I think it was in third grade I met Nancy Price down there at our condo creek. She was probably fishing but could have been doing anything. She was so in tune with nature and animals. We hung out at that creek all our summers long, fishing and gathering crawdads for later release. For 6 years. It was a heavenly spot with beautiful trees and places in the woods to hide and have fun. Once we went into the woods and found someone had a big hole in the ground where it appeared they had a club of sorts. I was terribly intrigued by this, and nervous they would catch us finding their hidey hole. 😊

So, sports? Nope, nope nope. I duz not do dem. I don't watch Superbowl or any of that stuff. It's on now I suppose, and I'm looking at the tv and listening to beautiful piano music. Rick is in his music room, playing. Things are peaceful.

There's no competition.

That's the big secret: I despise competition. I won't do it! If someone tries to compete with me, I will collapse in a useless heap, refusing to move a finger. I do not like it, no sir.

No clothing competition. I'm a frump. No Gotta-Look-As-Good-As-The-Neighbors. Nope. We're poor and that's that.

Now, board games and children's games? THAT was a different story!

I can get so excited playing a mental board game...like Scattergories or maybe a game of Charades...I cannot handle the excitement. I get so excited I get obnoxious.

Or Duck Duck Goose and 7-Up and all those games. What classroom games do you remember? The excitement was tremendous.

I've come to the conclusion my Thing is writing. Plus being a Dawnkey, and all that entails.

Enjoy the Super Bowl, sports fans.

Early Spiritual Beliefs

My first memories of what I perceived as God were as a very, very young child. It is a little yellow book called, "God Is Everywhere." This book was, and is, wonderful. I still recommend it for everyone as their first religious or spiritual book.

So, you see, my first impression of God was loving and goodness. He didn't have a name as far as I knew. He was simply God.

God loved us. God was impartial. God sat back and watched and took note.

I never made a connection between this and Santa.

I never lost my belief in Santa Claus.

Well, I sort of mean that. You see, my mother kind of manipulated me a bit. Sometimes it was keeping me compliant, another was by informing me that if I stopped believing in Santa, he would stop coming!!!

Horrors!

You can bet your butt I never had that Realization. Nobody ever surprised me.

Now, it's possible that I always knew. Always knew it was a put on that everyone believed in because it was fun and lovely and just wouldn't admit it. That would say impossible things about my childlike mind/brain.

Anyway. God was like an idea. A sweet, loving, comforting idea. He didn't become REAL to me until something very hokey, and very embarrassing happened. I saw a movie scene that moved me.

I can't tell you what it was. It's embarrassing. But it was a beautiful thing where it had previously been hate and ugliness. And things came to me, and I was filled with understanding of Things. This didn't happen until my 20s.

If I hadn't been "saved" at 11 or 12, I would think I'd just experienced salvation for the first time.

BTW, dad's mom, Grandma Camp, began trying to get me "saved," as in receiving salvation.

From what? I hear some of you wryly asking. From hell. Fiery, inferno-like hell burning you and screaming your guts out in intense agony for eternity. No breaks, no learning, no forgiveness, no nothing. You should have had faith and believed in God and Jesus when you were alive! Now it's too late! Muahahahah!!

I bought it hook, line and sinker.

I was terrified. I couldn't believe. I couldn't force myself to believe it. I was horribly afraid it was true though...I felt it must be true, but I still couldn't believe. I tried and tried, praying, to get salvation.

Grandma detected my lack of salvation and informed me I should go in the bathroom and get it done.

The salvation.

Get saved in that bathroom. Confess your sins and say truthfully you believe Christ died on the cross and rose up again and it was for your sins, and if you do not believe this, cannot believe this, will not believe this, whatever the case, you will GO TO BURNING FIERY HELL!

The Jack Chick Tracts didn't help.

Neither did Revelations.

And nighttime was scary. And that's what got dad's attention. He was furious. He had gone through the same thing as a child.

You might think that he would be sympathetic to me and sit me down and lovingly explain a kind loving God to me. You'd be wrong.

He was LIVID. I remember the screaming, the purple faced rage, the mocking of Jesus Christ, the jokes, sacrilegious jokes about God and Christ. It was horrid and it went on a while. Meaning a while that day, and many times in the future, and for then on for a long time.

I continued going to church with my grandmother! I insisted it was my own choice! I was hooked on the guilt and shame and fear.

I informed my grandmother I was saved around 11 or 12, when I made my many attempts, but not receiving any warm fuzzy feelings or light from the ceiling or whatever was supposed to happen when it... "worked."

That was irresponsible of her, sending me into a spiritual scary situation that way without warning me that there wouldn't necessarily be a "response."

Of course, I hear many of you saying it was irresponsible of anybody to tell someone they are going to hell if they don't believe Christ died on a cross and rose to save them.

So, that was my situation when I was around 12. I spent the next decade or so trying to deal with that. On and off through life I had the fear of hell at some level or another in the back of my spiritual mind.

I gradually got rid of it. I have spent my whole life shedding that early conditioning. I did it a little bit at a time.

WHAT I BELIEVE NOW

I don't have firm beliefs in anything.

I believe in God. I believe in the divinity of Christ. I believe in prayer, and invoke Jesus' name when praying.

I believe in the validity of everyone's personal path. An atheist's path is as valid as a Christian's or a Jew's or a Muslim's, for example.

These things I believe for me.

What you believe may vary.

You, e.g., might believe in several gods.

My belief does not trump your belief. I recognize I could be wrong.

Or maybe we're both right. And that is what I have come to say.

I love the story of the elephant and all the blindfolded people touch a different part of the elephant. (This could get comical and punny but I won't do that to you). They each have a different idea, according to their little chunk of understanding.

Everyone is learning. I don't believe I know one grain of sand in the ocean's worth of spiritual knowledge there is to learn.

Everyone has a valid path.

UNLESS.

There are unlesses.

When I say everyone has a valid path, I don't mean it's valid to murder someone for fun. When I say path, I mean like a spiritual or religious or atheist or whatever path.

OK, here's a list of some things I PREFER to believe. Doesn't mean I actively believe for certain, like I do that the sun will rise in the morning, just want to and choose to as best as possible.

   1. There is no burning, fiery hell. Unless it's for something demonic AND evil. And even then, I doubt it. I really doubt there's a burning hell out there somewhere on some plane, but I suppose it

could be real. What I don't believe is that my God created it and meant it to be for all those who reject salvation during their life on earth.

2. There will be a Dawnkey Island, if I want one. I believe when I die, I am going to be met by family and/or friend(s) who will help me pass over, where I will be processed for the next step, which will be either heaven, or reincarnation.

3. I believe we are all here to 1. Love and 2. Learn.

4. Atheists are treated the same as theists. They all cross over and get

processed and then talk with counselors who help them decide how to reincarnate or maybe they want to stay around a while. There might be a nasty Christian who hasn't done very well and will need to go back again and have some more learning experiences, while there might be a really good atheist who has been through the mill and learned all manner of soul growing experiences and done great things. Their guide will be happy with them.

5. Your experience may vary. What this actually means

is, literally, your experience in the afterlife may be different than mine.

6. Some people get stuck. For reasons. But it all comes out in the wash.

7. Hardship is not in vain. Everything you suffer through leaves an imprint on your psyche/soul and makes you what you are today.

8. Almost everybuddy has a guide. Maybe more than one. Meditate and ask your guide to tell you their name, and see if you can have the name come to you. It's fun. Try to relax and relax your mind and

not think, and see if a
name pops in your head.
Guides can help you.
Whether you believe in a
guide or a higher self,
same thing!

9. Relax every chance you
   get, from stress and strain.
   Unless you are exercising,
   and then, go to it. :D

10. LOVE EVERYBUDDY!
   Yeah, it all comes out in
   the wash, or how an old
   buddy used to say,
   "Everything's gonna be
   alright."

REINCARNATION-MY SECRET

I am going to go ahead and warn you with my headline. This is about as spiritual as it gets, so if you are turned off by such things you don't have to look.

I have a secret to share with you. This is going to take some bravery to share, but I have it!

I was fascinated by concentration camps at a very early age. I read The Hiding Place many times until I heard about Anne Frank and read that. It was kind of an obsession.

The obsession grew.

Soon, (like many other people I realize of course), I was believing that I was Anne Frank, reincarnated. I have a whole list of coincidences that I feel are significant, coincidences that I felt were put there by me on the other side, so that I would recognize who I was.

Anyway, I couldn't shake it. I could NOT SHAKE the idea that I was she.

I believed it up until the night before yesterday. Through thick and thin, crazy and sane, through the delusions and the clarity, my belief that I was Anne Frank continued.

It was embarrassing. Oh, yes...but I shared this with a handful of people, all of whom were very supportive.

But I have a good friend. A wonderful friend, who got me the spiritual information I needed.

I trust her implicitly. And she told me I was NOT Anne Frank.

Then she told me what made all the sense in the world to me: that I was similar in experience. I was a Jewish girl hiding from the Nazis.

It took me a full day to process it.

I got to thinking about all my "symptoms."

LIKE: eating like someone was going to take it away from me. Being terrified and praying several times a day, every day, hoping and praying that the police would not show up at my house and arrest me and take me away.

Being terrified to drive somewhere, for fear the police would get me.

I had no reason for these things.

There are other things.

Today, Rick and I went out. I caught myself doing a ritual type prayer to keep me from harm, and it occurred to me it wasn't necessary.

I went out into the sun, and rode in the car, and didn't fear. I felt ALIVE and FREE and able to do whatever I wanted! I even realized I could drive by myself and wouldn't be afraid! Maybe I will go out later and get some milk! By myself!

My life feels like something hugely significant happened.

I feel safe. And happy. And excited.

Who knows what I will be capable of now?

Out of the Funny Farm Into the Fire

Feb 12, 2010

Random ramblings from the recently released donkey (beware! Long rambling ahead!)

Some of you 'in the know' know about the expression I like to spread around: "Thanks for the fleas." This expression refers to Corrie Ten Boom's The Hiding Place, a story told about her experiences in a concentration camp. She tells of her sister Betsy's penchant for thanking God for ALL things. Corrie loses her temper and snarkily asks, "Even the fleas?"

Betsy says, yes! Let's thank Him for the fleas! And so, they did.

It came to their attention afterward that their Bible, the only source of hope and inspiration they had, was free from confiscation, because their barracks were flea ridden, and the guards wouldn't come in!

Yesterday (Wednesday) was a mixed bag of fleas. I'll get back to that later. I got out of Woodland Hospital on Tuesday around 1:30. I really wasn't ready to go. I knew I would have a big load of responsibilities waiting for me, the most pleasant of which would be contacting all the cheezfriends who had supported me. My family and I ended up wasting precious time going to Mercy

Medical for paperwork that wouldn't be ready until Wednesday. Then I had to go pay bills and run errands with deadlines. I had all sorts of nasty surprises awaiting me with my car, as my father and son tinkered with it. It is a '92 Acura with, I swear, what must surely be a poltergeist inside. Methinks said poltergeist was angered by their tinkering. Nuff sed...

Here's a synopsis of what happened to me and what I did, since January 27th.

Many of you know the dynamics of my relationship with my father. It is an extremely rare, to the point of shocking, occasion for me to talk back to him and get into an altercation. This is what happened. The details aren't important, or this post will never end. Suffice it to say that I quickly exploded out of control and into a rage, from all the suppression, and it was ugly. Of course, he did not see this as something to stop and analyze; he merely responded with cold fury.

I was so enraged with impotent fury that I went to my room and continued to drink. Eventually, late at night, drunk and in a tunnel vision (that means, dear friends and fellow Christians, that I had no thoughts of my family, including my son, or my cheezfrends, or God. I simply had a one-track mind and nothing else. Very scary...when the Bible says "...he who is deceived by it is not wise" that is not a ticket to drunkenness. It is a warning about the slippery slope that drunkenness is.) I pried off the blades of a disposable razor and cut my wrist.

It was harder than I suspected. I then thought about laying down on my arm and making it numb, and then cutting it. Thank God I was too impatient and angry to bother. I just let it slowly bleed and thought I would just go to bed and let it bleed out.

I awoke PO'd and severely angry to be alive. I finally went to the computer and started researching what I could do for help. I just knew it wasn't right to be doing this, but I didn't value myself enough to think I was worthy of going to the ER. It was a scary thought to go to the ER. I have never done anything like this before. I was afraid I'd be treated with derision and turned away. I have no money or insurance to pay that kind of bill. I knew calling an ambulance would awaken the household and might bring derision and anger and all manner of hysteria from my family. (No, I wasn't thinking clearly, but I can still imagine my father's face of disbelief and anger at the possibility of waking up to such a spectacle) So I got in the car and drove to the ER. At this point my wrist had a nasty cut in it, but it wasn't oozing, so that was no heroic feat.

They were so kind at the ER. I was immediately taken into the back and they had me in a room on a bed within a few minutes. I was to end up being there from about 8 am to 4:30 pm. I cried on and off all day. I was sad, numb, and felt hopeless. I was like a zombie.

Important note! If you ever go to ER and ask them to notify your family, don't. Ask for a phone and call them yourself. I asked them to notify mine, and was told okay, (by an unknowing soul, I'm sure) and then lay there for hours and hours expecting with doom to see their faces come around the corner, peering at me, as I lay there feeling smarmy from my incredibly selfish act. When they

didn't come, I started to wonder.
Finally in the afternoon, I asked
again and was told they don't
notify. I found out I could have a
phone brought to my room and
was told sure! And there was no
time limit! I immediately got a
hold of mom. I don't know why I
thought my mother would be
exasperated and disgusted with
me, but she was not, of course.
Maybe I thought it because I was
so tired of myself that I thought
she was, too. She was terribly
kind and warm. Unfortunately, it
was too late for them to get there
on time with anything for me
before I got transferred to
Woodland at 4:30. The techs
were so nice and friendly.
Everyone was. It was an eye-
opening experience. I figured

they could see my lame, wussy attempt at cutting myself and look at me with a pained, disgusted expression saying, "You are wasting our time. We are here for REAL victims, REAL patients, not the likes of your pathetic, whiny self." It was humbling to be treated so kindly by everyone.

They drove me to Woodland Hospital in Woodland, CA. It was embarrassing to be wheeled in strapped on a stretcher and knowing all the patients were checking me out. Again, I was met with much kindness. When I plainly (as I do, donkishly, lol) told them the chair was too small for my big butt, and I needed another chair without arms, the sweet tech started talking about

how tall I was (I'm only 5'5 ½",
but she was tiny,) as if to say, oh,
you're not fat, you're tall. Such a
sweet lady.

The next day my family came. I
felt awkward. Not much smiling.
Still zombie like. I think mom was
kind of stunned. It truly was a
strange thing for me to do. Sean
was his normal, serious-faced
self. Dad was subdued and polite.
He did not appear to be drunk.
They brought me things.

Never during my stay did I ever
feel that taboo feeling of being in
a psych ward, or afraid of it. I just
cocooned and felt taken care of
and calm.

Sometimes I cried and was
depressed, but it got better.

The food was wonderful and plentiful, and the staff and patients came to care for me.

They diagnosed me with depression, bipolar disorder, and gave me Antabuse. Those three meds have me knocked for a loop. I'm always sleepy, and I'm confused, too. I am unable to think of simple things sometimes. I haven't gone back to work yet. I am stressing over that. I don't know if I can. I'm a courier. Calling the doctor tomorrow to talk about THAT problem.

I didn't miss the alcohol when I was in there. Don't really miss it now, either. Isn't that strange?

While in the hospital I called work and was told this coworker, a girl I feel like a mother or sister to, a very young married mom with 2 small kids, had lost her husband. He died of a brain aneurysm. His funeral was when I was in the hospital. She had no idea why I didn't come to it. I was devastated. I called her and cried and explained what happened and how sorry I was. He was the only goodness in her life, I think, besides her kids. How incredibly heartbreaking. I keep thinking about Valentine's Day and how hideous it will be for her. There is always someone else to make you realize what a whiner you are being. What can I say to her? I am at a loss.

Wednesday, I spent approximately 4 hours messing around with a Medical like office.

You'd think I'd be about crazy. I filled out the form wrong, and basically was an idiot. Poor clerk. I was very calm though, then started crying at some point (before the paperwork fiasco) for no discernable reason. Just sat there and the tears poured down. That's what it's been like. This crazy behavior.

Coming home I thought about my cheezfrends, and how much they love me and support me and what a heinous, selfish thing I'd done. And I realized even given that, they loved me anyway. Then for the first time, the enormity of God's same kind of love struck me and I felt like a worm. I began verbally accosting myself and crying.

I started questioning my good works. I decided I was a coward who did good deeds because subconsciously I am afraid of punishment and I think being good will keep me out of trouble, not because I am a good person. I basically ripped myself several new orifices on the way home, howling all the way.

Then I decided to throw melodramatic attention whore into the mix, and that I was beating myself up so I could get my melodramatic spike fix. I was doomed. I could think of no good intentions, no purity of motive to defend myself. By the time I got home I was exhausted from the self-attack and its resulting confusion.

That's what I'm going through. It is very selfish. I need the positive feedback, yet I feel guilty about it.

I am staying hopeful for when the meds kick in. Right now, I'm just kind of feeling strange.

More later if I think of it.

Thank you to all who sent love and concern, and posted and emailed. I love you all so much. You help get me through. Bless you and yours.

Valentine's- A Mixed Bag

I remember Valentine's Days with satisfied happiness. The memories are good.

Just as I said that I remembered a terrible Valentine's Day.

I had to fire someone on Valentine's Day, and I didn't realize it was even that holiday, unTIL she burst into horrible, hot tears and informed me they had great plans, and needed the money, and so forth and so on. It was most terrible and I felt like the Biggest S#!t in the universe. Maybe I was.

I wasn't used to firing people. Usually, the owner did that. I'm sure he didn't trust me.

I always thought of Valentine's Day to be for anyone from anyone, that it is a day of LOVE and not just romantic love but familial love and platonic and all that. I loved giving Valentine's presents and cards to my family. To have to fire someone on a day like that...it's so sad. I hope she was able to bounce back quickly and find a much better job.

OK, moving on.

I am sure my family and friends have given me many wonderful Valentines over the years. Most, I would say, of my V experience has probably been non-romantic, and that suits me just fine.

I never did experience much romance and magic on Valentine's Day. It just wasn't meant for me to receive much romantically on that day. I guess what is Meant to Be is for me to GIVE it every V Day. Which I enjoy thoroughly.

I do remember a present from my ex, though. The most beautiful pewter wand. It had gemstones on the ends, and was pewter with vines and such swirling round the wand, and it was stunning. Something else came with it too...and sadly I can't remember what that was. I still have the wand, sitting on a shelf with crystals and such, which is significant because I lost so much in the move from Midwest to CA.

My parents would always buy me candy and cards and they would be sitting on the dining room table waiting for us, in the morning, along with mine to them. Valentine's Day was pleasant every year with them, boyfriend or not, and mom would invariably make a nice meal for us. She was like a Martha Stewart with much color and vibrancy and excitement.

A few times I would buy dad a Romeo and Juliet cigar and maybe a small bottle of luxury spirits or what have you. Something like that. He was HARD to buy for. I bought him a *lot* of beautiful lighters over the years. One year I bought him a Spongebob Squarepants pair of boxers. They said, "NO MORE MR. NICE GUY" I doubt if he ever wore them, but when he saw them, he actually kind of grinned. That was enough from him to make me extremely happy. There was a special grin he had for really special moments. I saw that grin in a picture of him at my first wedding, to Tony. He was so refreshingly happy, that big clear grin on his face. The day he died, Thanksgiving last year, I was sitting at the table after he passed, and suddenly saw his face in my vision: it was that same Special Grin and I knew he was seeing his friends on the other side and was happy. And that made everything alright.

Valentine's Day was almost always GOOD and happy and fulfilling. I always felt loved on Valentine's Day.

Did you celebrate V Day in elementary school? We were allowed to decorate white sacks and hang them up. Or something. I remember with great excitement the bulging sacks the popular kids got. It was quite interesting to wonder what wonderful goodies their loving friends had given them. I had a bit of wistfulness, wishing *I*, too, would get such lumpy wonders, but I was satisfied to get the little V cards like everyone else did. It was so exciting.

There was a boy I had a crush on. I had forgotten about him. It was kindergarten, I believe? Or second grade? His name was George. I thought he was amazingly handsome. I think he had green eyes and dirty blonde hair. He gave me a light bulb picture on a V card and it said, "You turn me on!" I had that Valentine Mod-Podged on a little wooden board and mom helped me. I had it for years. I was like that.

I looked him up years later and called him on the phone. I was 11-14. Somewhere in there. It was so brave of me. It was a terrible call. I made a fool of myself.

Ah, the things we remember. Yet I adore Valentine's Day. I am always loving everybuddy and this is the best day besides Christmas to do it.

I wish the happiest, peacefulest, most wondermuss day for you. I hope you are rolling in love and

happies. and if you aren't, know
that I love you and you are
special.

The Marlboro Man and the Bed Stealer

I used to work in the home health care field. I have tremendous respect for nurses' aides and home health aides. It's exhausting, often thankless work for usually not very good pay. You really must have your heart in it. Those who don't, have no business doing this work. I've had so many funny, touching, and memorable experiences working in this field. Here is one of the highlights:

Mr. L liked to smoke. Oh, did he like to smoke. Being that his home was a convalescent center, though, this was not a common treat for him. He was reduced to smoking at certain breaktimes. He also got one beer a day. You can certainly appreciate any opportunity to smoke was met with a quickness to the breakroom.

The Bed Stealer liked to steal beds. It mattered not whose. He was not a particular man. Any old bed would do, besides his own. The bed was always snoozier on the other side of the hall.

The Bed Stealer was not a dull man. No, he was quite bright, apparently, for one day, when faced with the lack of enticing beds, he hatched a plan.

Now, I do not know if the Bed Stealer had happened upon this room and decided he liked the look and feel of this particular bed, or was just getting some particular glee out of twerping this particular victim, but he set his eye on...The Marlboro Man.

He informed the M.M., "They're smoking in the breakroom."

Sweeter words never spoken. Oh, evil Bed Stealer!!

Imagine this man, shuffling along the corridor, eyes as intense as eagles, the door at the end of the corridor his salvation.

"Smoking...smokin the breakroom....breakroom...they're smokin...in the...smokin in the...they're smoking in the...they're smokin..." he mumbled to himself as he went down the hall.

I was not there when the M.M. entered the breakroom, nor was I there, to see the expression and response at the cold, heartless response, "No, Mr. L., no one is smoking."

I can only imagine very vividly, what transpired when a highly infuriated Mr. L returned to his room and found the Bed Stealer– the Liar!!!– WALLOWING! in his bed.

Shall we mercifully close the curtain on this scene?

March 21, 2008

Anger

I got mad the other day.

Not just angry, crazy.

I was riding along coming home and noticed someone on my butt. This used to drive me crazy but somehow, I lost notice of it at the last moment and made a right curve to pull in on the left: they tried to pass me.

I slammed on the brakes and lost it.

Where you feel like you're watching yourself. I was shrieking like a madwoman. They ended up driving on past. I pulled in my driveway and got inside and realized they know where I live now, and I became mildly concerned, for the first time, that they could be angry and come back later and do something. They could even be a close neighbor.

I pondered all this and thought about the contrasts of my rage and my normal dull passivity of emotion.

How can I feel so dull and also have such bouncy highs? Writing seems to be the stimulus that gets me going. When I write things that are meant to be loving, I become very emotional.

There is a time and a place for anger.

I'm not using it properly.

It's coming to my attention that maybe I shouldn't be as calm as

I've been...that being emotionally calm isn't a great thing to aspire to. This may not seem logical, but: I haven't become calm, I've become dully passive at times. I feel like the last 5 years have been of huge significance to me. I feel that the last presidency term caused me so much distress that I internalized it. So has repeatedly losing friends and family. (Deaths, I mean) And, hugely, my father's decline in health.

It's not good for me to internalize stuff. I need to speak my mind, in written form, and get it out. That's what I do.

I'm in the wilderness now, with this subject. I don't know what is going on with me, but I need to figure out what it is, and express myself rationally and logically.

Except, that's not what I really do well. What I really do well is emote. (I use emote, which is often associated with an actor, but not always. I want to make this distinction because my desire is transparency, and I would hate if anyone thought I was "acting" or "fake.") So, yeah, I tend to show emotion in a theatrical manner, and I might have learned in my household not to show anger.

That just reminded me that I've always associated humor with anger.

I remember being very young and reading Mad Magazine and loving the characters' drawings. I think it was Al Jaffee that thrilled me first. His hefty round female figures prancing along on pointy feet amused me to no end. When he drew an enraged person, I was beside myself with laughter. I found rage to be *explosively* funny. I, of course, was not permitted to be enraged. I was told at an early age by mom that when I felt the need, I could scream into a pillow.

Dad would rage, mom would be calm and listen and try to apply emotional balm, and my guts would churn.

I twisted this somehow, because I came to find angry, impotently furious people hilarious. But only if they couldn't hurt me! If there was any way they could punish me for laughing at them, I wouldn't be laughing.

I have a horrible, horrible shame at something I did when I was little.

My cousin had to have some kind of leg device(s) on him when he slept. He was in his room screaming in distress over his imprisonment, and I was wriggling with glee and laughter in my bed in the other room.

His mother looked at me and smiled the kindest smile, and said, "You don't like him very much, do you?"

Well, I was mortified, of course, as I should have been. I felt sickened at what I had done. I

DID like that boy. I found him adorable.

Here's what I think happened, now that I'm writing about it. I think he was expressing what I was not allowed to express, and I felt glee about that. I wasn't happy that he was sad, it was something else. It was an act of fury and unleashed frustration, something I would never have been allowed to do.

I was safe in bed, with no one hurting me, listening to someone yell, and nothing was going to happen to me because of it. I did not have to worry that someone would come into my room and get me. I don't know why I would worry about this.

This is my only thought of how I can explain what I did. I feel horrid about it.

I just realized something else: about the time I lost my anger I lost my sense of humor.

Today I amused myself gigantically: Terry said KNOCK KNOCK, as precedes a joke, and I decided to write, "I know it's you Terry" and this sent me into peals of laughter. It was weird to be laughing so much.

Joking about disguising oneself may be stressful to me...I remember a horrific nightmare where Superman was bald, in the shower. I was terrified. This, I suppose, said to me that someone was misrepresenting themself.

That scares me.

Now I've noticed my eyes are wide. I'm getting into scary psychological territory here.

When I was 14, I watched "Play Misty for Me" with Clint Eastwood. I had never seen a horror movie. This was NOT horror. It was...kind of a romantic thriller I suppose. Anyway, Jessica Walter, if that was her name[4], had black hair, like my dad. She was a terror in the movie. After the movie, I was freaked out and mom came into my room to be with me while I dressed for bed. Dad, wanting to check on me, decided to peek his

____

[4] Editor's note: It was.

head around the door to take a look. I saw his black hair and made the association and lost it. I LEAPED up on the bed and screamed and screamed and screamed.

I hold stuff within.

I suspect I am holding much in. How I get into that, I will leave for the next paper.

ANGER PART II: HOLDING IT IN

I've no idea where to begin.

I've been holding it in all my life.

As I told you before, when I was in a baby bed, I would hold my breath and pass out from the yelling in the apartment.

I watched my father emote for 56 years. And I wasn't supposed to act that way.

Something happened though, when I was about 14.

I remember so clearly where we were standing. I was standing in front of the closet, listening to him interrogate and yell at me. I don't remember what for.

You hear that? I don't remember what for. What good did it do to have a fit when I don't even remember what I did wrong.

Once, not long ago, I explained he was crying wolf.

But back to the story. He was grouching along, and I had this thought in my head: KISS OFF ASSHOLE. This is not language or the kind of expression that appealed to me. I found it crude and a turn off. I hated that it was in my head.

I was listening respectfully and watching with reserve when all of a sudden...omg...

It came out of my mouth.

I, the social wuss of the century, said KO AHOLE to my father.

His face sank. Mine, I am sure, was priceless.

I was so horrified I didn't even apologize—I just stared, waiting for my punishment.

He turned and left and never said another word about it.

Later I talked to mom about it. She said he came to her, and said, "Can you believe she said that?"

And her response?

"Well, Frank, you were probably worrying the hell out of her." I can hear her calmly saying that in my mind.

Holding in anger is dangerous. Because it can seep out or explode.

I remember being bullied one day at the lockers, and a sudden explosion coming out of me. I HOWLED. They were terrified and probably ran. An adult was fetched. I don't remember a lot after that.

So, yeah, I hold things in and am apt to explode.

I don't have many angry episodes to share, because I was never a person who was comfortable expressing anger.

I'm afraid if I get angry, I will lose control.

What are some other thoughts on anger?

I should be angry at some people, and I'm not. At least it doesn't feel like I am.

The woman who interfered with my relationship with my first husband. She was an asshole. Yes, an asshole. She had redeeming qualities, but she was bound and determined to be disrespectful of me.

I ended up living with her, in a situation that was insane.

Once I came home to my bedroom and found vomit all over my bed. I was informed her guest did this after she fed him spaghetti. I was expected to clean up the mess myself.

What good does it do to become angry?

Well, sometimes it helps. Sometimes it stops a bully.

Sometimes I was afraid, and had to *pretend* to be angry to stop the crap.

I'm struggling here to express.

Do I have anger that is pressed so far down inside I can't get it out? I thought I had gotten rid of all that. I thought I had worked on this. I thought it was gone.

But now, I can't seem to even GET angry.

Horrible things are happening. Right now. Arizona just passed a law saying you can't video the cops. Am I angry? No. Just tired.

But let someone do something petty and irritating, and maybe I'll explode.

It's frightening. What is my rage capable of doing? What kind of trouble will I get in?

I find myself trying to psychically predict what will happen in a situation, and getting mad thinking about the possibilities when nothing has even happened yet.

I'm dancing around the subject but don't know how to get into it.

I'll meditate and see if I can think of a time I was really angry.

Sometimes I shake when I'm angry, and the feeling is so overpowering I cannot express it smoothly and politely. I hate this feeling.

Ah, a petty act. A petty act can make me LIVID. I don't know why this is so. I can put up with all manner of atrocities until someone gets petty with me.

"Say Puh." That was the headline on my email.

Some context? Well, I was dating a man who had something wrong that caused him to walk in a severely affected manner. I cannot remember what was wrong. He was dishonest by not informing me of his disability, for lack of a better word. I watched him walk toward me in the parking lot and thought, "Why didn't he tell me? I wouldn't have cared." Anyway, in one of my letters I later wrote to him, I said, "I say PUH!" meaning, I pooh-pooh the idea that his disability would cause me to not be interested.

So, he writes me a letter. I don't see it at first.

I get another, and its title? "Say Puh."

He thought I had ghosted him because I didn't answer his first letter. And assumed if I had, it would be because of his disability. Not because of anything about his personality! Nope, must be the disability.

This infuriated me. When I saw the petty "Say Puh" needling, it made my blood boil.

He was a neat guy. He sang Rocky Raccoon for me and played the guitar. And bought for me a bottle of some kind of liquor.

I was a raging drunk and drank it all.

When he discovered this, he ghosted ME.

He just decided I was a drunk. That's cool. I totally understood that.

But then later there was a kerfluffle. He wanted to have his cake and eat it too.

See, he wanted to tell me that he wasn't going to see me because of my drinking, but when I ACCEPTED this, and told him he was probably right, that's when he got butthurt.

I ended up being e-screamed at by a platonic friend of his who was supposed to be fixing his computer situation and went through his mail and decided I would rather be an alcoholic than date her friend, who, I was informed, HAD PLENTY OF OTHER WOMEN TO CHOOSE FROM. She repeatedly tried to pound this into my head.

FINE. I do not care.

Puh.

I fear that I do not get angry enough at atrocities. When I read about things or see them in the news, it just deepens my despair. It doesn't anger me, it just further exhausts and saddens me. I am afraid this is happening to ALL of us.

What is going to become of us?

It appears Russia is going to invade Ukraine. How can this be?

How can we allow such an act? One little emoting donkey cannot stand up to the world and say WTF ARE YA DOIN??? And have a reasonable response.

I'm not getting anything accomplished here. This is supposed to be a process paper. I think I know what that means, maybe not. I'm supposed to be figuring out my anger problems here. This is usually how I work my majick. By writing. Except it's not working.

I can be cruel. I can get SO ANGRY, so cold. Revenge is best served cold. I don't like revenge. Revenge sickens me.

There was a guy I'd been seeing. I was his girlfriend. This was a fact.

Well, the subject came up, and he had the nerve to inform me I was not, in fact, his girlfriend.

This did not sit well with me.

I thought and thought about it. Cold anger.

I cut him off, and shut down the Candy Shop, so to speak. For TEN YEARS.

He called me every other day for what felt like over a month, leaving messages. Eventually he said he loved me. I knew it was bullshit. I enjoyed those calls. I enjoyed feeling powerful.

For ten years I held that grudge.

Why can't I get mad like a normal person? Why don't atrocities infuriate me? Is it because I can't do anything about them? That I don't want to feel badly if I cannot make it stop?

I'll tell you why I'm mad at him.

I know the answer.

It was pettiness.

It was a conversation about theft. I disagreed with his brother, who was a psychiatrist. He had stated that thievery was learned, not innate. I asked my boyfriend, who taught my son to steal?

No answer.

He smugly held his belief, and this infuriated me. I, for some reason, felt superior in my belief and was angry at him for not siding with me.

Can you believe that?

I think that is what drove my anger.

What's wrong with me?

WHIPPERSNAPPERS

What's the world coming to?
Why, when I was a little wee
dawnkey, if you got

in a man's yard, he'd beat you
within an inch of your life with a
rake, a hoe, a

board with a rusty nail in it, hell,
whatever he could get his hand
on. My old

papaw'd take his belt off'n
beatcha half dead right there on
mainstreet while

the cops ate their pie in
Woolworths. Nowadays they
don't do squat. I saw five

hooligans FIVE jackassing
around in old man Thubburt's
yard. ooooooo if I'd

had a ballpeen hammer I would
have laid into the little
lollygaggers. But I had

groceries

to carry in.

RACIST

My dad was raised to be a racist.

His father was a southern fundamentalist Baptist preacher. His mother played the piano for the church, amongst other things.

They were terribly racist.

They taught it to dad.

Dad said when he was little, he heard his dad talking to his mother. He said he had had her "checked out" and she had "black blood" in the family. She asked him what he was going to do, as they had two children. He said he didn't know. Apparently, nothing came of it as they remained together until Grandpa's death.

But the relationship was never the same.

This would have been in the late 40s or the 50s that this happened. Grandpa was born in 1911 and died at the age of 50, so that would have been in '61. I was born 4 years later.

Despite the racism, dad worshipped his father. Grandpa never hit him. Never. Years later dad would cry and whisper this to me. He said once when his mother insisted he get a beating, his father took him into the bathroom. He hit the belt on the wall. Then he said something like, you might want to start crying. He was faking the beating so grandma would be satisfied.

He remembers wondering why his parents wouldn't let the black man working for them eat with them at the dining table, instead of out on the back porch step.

He remembers lots of things.

He tried to overcome it. He had a best friend who was black. This does not mean that he got a "Get out of racism free" card. But it was eye opening for him. He was brought into his friend's family and friend's circle. It meant so much to him. He paid for his friend to go through Xray school, and his friend paid back every penny.

In the last few years, he found another black friend here in Sacramento. He thought he was close to him- enough to tell him a bad joke.

Yes, bad is a euphemism. For you-know-what. I was appalled. I didn't understand how he could do something so dumb. His friend never forgave him or saw him again.

It tore him up. He'd cry in front of me about it.

He learned so much, but still had so far to go. Did it make a difference?

My racist grandma, his mother, had 4 grandchildren. Three girls including me, and her grandson. Both girls besides me, married black men and had lots of black children. We have lots of black people in our family.

FYI- this does not give me a Get Out of Racism Free card, either. Just because I have black folks in my family doesn't make me free of stupidity. I still can make mistakes and misunderstand things. I will never be perfect, but I still try really hard to do the right things.

Grandma lived with one of her grandchildren. She asked one of her great grandchildren "What does it feel like to be black?" She still used the N word up until I don't know how long.

Grandpa, the man that dad adored, died at 50. Grandma died at 100. Dad couldn't understand why... why he lost his dad whom he idolized, and his mom, who was mean to him, lived another

50 years. He grieved horribly for him.

I think he was still grieving when he died.

He remembered things. Horrible things.

He was the preacher's son. "You think you're better than us!" He was small, short. He got beaten up. When he got home, he was beaten by his mom for being in a fight. He was always the new kid, and got beaten up for that, too.

He grew up angry with a chip on his shoulder.

When he started a new high school, he finally got fed up. Someone came up to him and bullied. People circled around yelling "fight."

And. He. Did.

He kicked that bully's ass. They became friends. Dad became popular and was class Valedictorian.

When he married mom, he did a lot of screaming and yelling. I don't think he could help it. Mom said I would cry and pass out when he did this.

He was so unhappy. Mom tried so hard. She made everything perfect. She treated us like gold. She made a beautiful warm nest for us and tried to be so happy.

He was the best provider ever. And hard worker. And brilliant and talented. Best woodworker I ever saw. He was such a perfectionist. He was so valued at work that when he tried to leave to make more money, they gave him a 50% pay raise and a new title to justify it.

I understand he passed over, to the other side. I also understand he is back at times...doing little jobs and work and things there and checking on mom so when she passes he can help her cross over.

Sean dedicated "My Way" to dad. This made dad cry. Lots of things made dad cry near the end.

He's happy and free of his burdens. That makes my heart soar.

That was the Mayan doomsday date.

It was also the date of my insanity attack.

Every year, on social media, I am reminded of my anniversary posts. So, every December I get posts from every December from last year all the way back. That's a lot of rubbing of a Dawnkey's nose in something. It's pretty embarrassing, frankly.

Why should I be embarrassed for being psychotic? Well, because it was my own fault. I knew what would happen if I went off my medication, but I did it anyway. All for the Mighty Bipolar High.

Except I really had no idea how psychotic I would become. It was frightening and horrible.

I am going to try to recapture what happened by examining my emails and by examining what memories I have now.

Wednesday December 26, 2012

"These concepts are represented visually by mathematical boxes. with three axes in them. For the male side, there is A, B, and C (the names are not listed here) There is a female side, too. And a spiritual. I sense these all add up to 666, and I am going to be responsible for causing this opening in the veil and letting it in, something I have to be knowledgeable through karma to be able to do. But the polarity is that it feels evil. But doing so will allow an end, and so we can all return to God.”

“I disagree. I want out.

My grandmother called it sideways, I just found out a year or so ago. She is such a derp. But I found out she went through menopause and wanted to kill herself. Wonder if she had the same experience and our time placements are looping each other.”

To my friend A, I thought he was hypnotized and I was trying to get him “saved.”

I found an email to him that said, “You will never be hypnotized again and you will reject all past hypnotizing attempts.

You will understand what I am telling you and not be dissuaded.

HUH?"

More weirdness I found in emails:

- I think I have a new revelation. I think time used to be linear and when time travel was discovered it caused an endless looping, much like the polarities of the inner and outer spiraling of the Fibonacci shell. This realization is what my mind is trapped in, flipping back and forth and causing me to need to take a side and stick with it to avoid becoming crazy.

- So my question is, how do I get rid of this new awareness so I can go back to normal? When the meds kick in in about a week or so, maybe?

- Mom always said, "You cannot become sensitive until you become aware of coarseness." See, I always thought innocence WAS sensitive. But I see it isn't. Losing that one locus and it becoming more than one dimensional is what is f ing with me and making me loopy, if you'll excuse the pun. I cannot deal with it intellectually.

- Just like floating is not flow!!!! O.O It's like a four-dimensional locus!!!!

When you try to post something and it doesn't post, is that someone traveling back in time and thwarting it, until you post something different?

- I fear I will be trapped in a locus (hell) to stabilize this paradigm. Maybe this is what causes some schizos to think they are God.
And maybe this is why the universe has to lie to people and tell them not to kill themselves or they will go to hell or be stuck in an endless cycle of karma, because otherwise everyone will just kill themself and go back to heaven, ruining the fun of the Game.

There was book I've been
searching for for years. I read
it as a child. Something
about The Game of Life and
someone named Gregory and
it involved chess, I think. I
have a queer feeling this is
related.
If innocence is the center of
coarseness and sensitivity,
then what is the center of
going with the flow and flow?
I sense that is the last key to
be unlocked that will truly
even me out with your
balanced nature and stop
this all.

- Yes, but this experience is
  not good. I feel like I am in a
  hell of sorts right now. What
  I am experiencing is surreal

and unpleasant.
I don't have the inner calm you do to deal with it as you do.
I'm probably hooked up to a damned machine and being experimented on by some group. *eyeroll*
Yeah, and you're on the reality side of it, communicating with me.
So, if I take the red pill, can I wake up? Or maybe click two red pills together and say "There's no place like B's laboratory?" *smile*
This would also explain why I see "holes" in the fabric. I chalk it up to hormones."

And another:

"It's too long and drawn out.

I have spiraled inward like a shell, and I see parallels in everything. Everything. It's like a wrong decision was made and I have to fix it so the world will be different."

There are so many. It just goes on and on and on and ON.

Another:

"Remember AP? I said he was in the Intelligence and I think he did something to us

one time he went inside the building and left dad outside and dad thought he saw a spaceship but never told anyone

I said he should tell AP....

he was gonna call him and decided against it.

I think he DID call him and AP made him forget.

Also, AP talked dad into being interested in Amway once but dad got over it.

Now check out Amway.... a cult?

Amway screwed with me and C, too.... come to think of it, and I remember the guy of the pair was named R and looks exactly like this creepy R on my other FB who did weird shit!!!!

This is exhausting. I need to quit spiraling and do something.

Do you have a prisoner locked up that you could release? I sense that could be the KEY here."

Reading all this gives me a headache.

Absolute insanity, if anyone doubted it before.

This is what it was like to be insane.

I'm sharing this with you in this way because it's the most severe example of my psychosis and I truly want everyone to understand how serious it was.

Sometimes I think people think I sit at home on my butt and don't do anything to contribute to society. There is a reason I have a diagnosis of schizo-affective. Now I'm getting into a new subject I should tackle on a different essay.

Back to psychosis.

I remember thinking mom and dad were Mrs. and Mr. God. I somehow thought I had been reincarnated again and again, and was Eve, was Mary, I wasn't even sure which, was the Mona Lisa, and Anne Frank. There was no logic involved.

At one point I was convinced I was thinking in binary. This was the deepest hell I experienced. I cannot explain to you why I felt this was so hellish, just that it was so. Hell doesn't have to be burning. It can be mental hell, too.

I remember the day the police came.

I just remembered the watch. The pocket watch our friend gave me for Christmas. It was a lovely gold or brass colored pocket watch. She had attached a glorious octopus on the front and a ruby colored crystal in the center! It was amazing! She also gave me, and I just remembered this, a kind of round shaped container for beads. I was convinced it was a tesseract and if I recall correctly, I thought the watch would help me time travel. I was thrilled with her thoughtfulness at these gifts. I am sure she took my over exuberance as just my natural excitement when I am given a gift.

Back to the Police Day. I remember that I had it in my head that our friend Art was pulling a Manchurian Candidate deal on my dad, and calling him and hypnotizing him, basically.

Now stop for a minute and think about how ludicrous this is. How could dad be God and also be tricked and hypnotized by Art? It made no sense. No one was there to question me though, because they did not know these crazy thoughts.

So I went and got Dad's phone and REMOVED THE BATTERY!! And HID IT!!

Now this may not seem like such a big deal, but if you've read about our relationship, you'd understand that normally I would have to be out of my mind to do something like that to my father's property.

And. I. Was.

Dad was very anal about the phones. He quickly discovered his missing phone.

I cannot remember if he shouted my name and beat on my door when he discovered the missing phone. I may have stayed in there a bit, causing him alarm. At any rate, I finally answered my bedroom door, and I matter of factly explained what I had done, and why.

At some point they also found out I had stabbed my c-pap machine's computer chip.

I had taken a sword off my wall and decided that I was saving the world. I cannot remember the exact details. I remember at some time, lying in bed at night, and thinking somehow evil could see me, and I had to remain in the dark. I somehow did something in the dark, and it may have been the stabbing of the chip, while thinking someone was watching. It was terrifying. I did this, brought on this terror, because I thought I had to save the world.

I would say when I explained to my dismayed mother what I had done, that is probably when they called the doctor. The doctor, in turn, said to call the police.

The police were nice. I was shockingly un-terrified. In fact, I was exasperated and informed them they should take a look at my father's room, with all the knives covering the walls. They sort of glossed over this suggestion. They were kind and courteous and said I could go to the hospital with them or my parents, so I chose my parents.

I really should have been hospitalized. I was not. What happened next even astounded the great big ole hospital aide who was there to protect the situation. (i.e., when I started to get annoyed, he was THERE)

My father was terrified to watch me snap at the doctor and tell her not to touch me, I believe. I did not like this doctor, did not trust her, and felt very paranoid.

I sat on the gurney and begged my mother not to let them take me away. I was afraid. I didn't know what I was afraid of.

I convinced both my mother and doctor to give me a pill and let me take it. The aide kept saying over and over he'd never seen anybody come in like that and then get to go back home. I kept saying, knowingly, because, being delusional, I felt all special and important, "I know," "I know."

I do not know why they trusted me so, but they gave me the pill and I drank, but managed somehow or another to let it stick in my mouth until I got outside in the car. I slowly and very carefully unpacked it from my mouth. Some had dissolved. I would take the medication as I promised her, but not that day. That day I was terrified of what the medication would do to me.

I want to impress on you all that none of this had to make sense to me. I was in a psychotic fog. I was not reasoning properly. I thought Jesus was my brother.

Maybe I got that part right.

Seems to me that those three things should all be different papers. Books, in fact. But I don't have the ability to write books on those subjects.

I do have the ability to rant, Andy Rooney style, and that is what I shall do.

This book is going to be set in the time of COVID and Trump, and it seems fitting that I should write about how this historic mess affects and has affected me.

The "DEATH" part is, of course, the family and all the friends I've lost in the last few years.

Seems like the last 5 years have been the worst and the best. So many times now, I have quoted those words, "It was the best of times, it was the worst of times."

Thanksgiving, 2021, my father passed.

A bunch of friends have passed. Some have contacted me from the dead.

But mostly there's the slow, terrible trudge of time in which people kept fighting and arguing and getting sick and dying. And all in the meantime, was Trump.

He tore my guts up. Him. Turtle-face McConnell. Linsy whatcha callit. Lindsay Graham?

Today I saw the news. It said Arizona has passed a law that the cops can't be videotaped.

OMGOMGOMGOMG

Do right wing people know what horror that strikes in me/us?

I don't think, if I had kept a diary all this time, these last four years, that it would have been possible to express in such a long drawn-out way, what I can express in this essay, and that is: I think we as a world/nation have PTSD.

Now I know some people have it from, say, the Vietnam war. That's sacrosanct. But I think it has milder cases, and I think collectively we have it.

I haven't given it a lot of psychological thought so I don't know if it's true or not.

I feel different feelings. Partly I am overwhelmingly happy

spiritually. Also, I feel numb. But I am still intellectually and morally intact.

Russia is invading Ukraine.

Those poor people. Why aren't we helping them? Why isn't anybody helping them fight them off? What the hell has happened to us? Why aren't we putting a stop to this?

I'm only one little Dawnkey in a mute world. A world that is sitting by and watching Ukraine get invaded.

I just said a prayer for Ukraine. I started to cry, and it got ugly. I didn't know I had that in me.

I really didn't know.

It was like a quick and violent shower. All I can do now is sit back and pray. I don't even have any money to send to anyone, if it would even do any good. I used to like to give money and gifts to people who needed it. Now our budget has changed, and I don't have the funds anymore. At least I felt like I was doing my tiny little part, but now, nothing. All I have to share is my words with you.

And prayer.

I feel so bad when people put others down for praying. Sometimes it's all we have to give, and we give it our all.

COVID is just the never-ending bleh. It appears the rules about wearing masks inside have been lifted. I could shop in Walmart without a mask, if I so chose. I don't think it's going to be over any time soon.

People won't wear masks and won't cooperate and THEY are the reason we KEEP having to wear the masks. GRRR!!!

Seems that I should give you a mental picture of me here.

I sit at a table with a computer at it, next to a window. There is usually sun outside, as it is sunny California, USA. *Smiles here* I have beautiful forest green velvet lined drapes that I am so pleased and proud of, hanging in front of the big front windows facing the street. The street is only about four feet from the window. If I choose to open my drapes I have beautiful rose bushes with coral red roses, huge blooms. They are deliciously fragrant.

I live in a mobile home park. Everybody is very close to one another, and you can hear all the outside noises.

In front of me is the couch, then a green Oriental rug, and then a beautiful fireplace lit up with lights from my friend Nancy. A giant starry night picture done in aqua and orange on the fireplace, instead of the requisite television. And a television to the right of the fireplace.

It's a pleasant place. I love my spacious home and am very happy here with Rick.

We are hermits.

We both hate to go out, especially to drive, or walk, or anything. We are homebodies. Going out makes us nervous.

How do I spend my days? Well, sometimes I do a little housework. Sometimes I make efforts to read. I rarely watch television. Mostly I am on the internet, sitting at the table, typing away.

What do I do when I'm on the internet?

I am kind to people.

That's it. That's my Universal Job. To analyze and write things down, and to be kind to people. I spend my days and nights writing and looking for people in distress.

People in distress.

Whatever kind of distress it is.

I've been friends with all kinds of people. NO ONE escapes my love.

Nobuddy.

I am able to love the most unloveable.

But that doesn't mean I like everybuddy. I love them, but only some people I have feelings of like. I love my friends, but I also like them.

I try to love Trump, but I don't like him.

And I refuse to hate him.

Oh, has he baited us to do so. He has been responsible for horrible things. There are so many I don't know where to begin. And it isn't necessary. Plenty of history books will tell the tale of this man.

Plenty of diaries, too, I imagine.

But probably not a lot of schizo affective disordered people who are Dawnkeys, telling how they came to love everybuddy.

BTW, I'll tell you how: when I joined ICHC and started loving those people, it came to be that when I'd see a stranger I felt wary of? I'd just say to myself, what if that was a cheezfrend? And my attitude would change.

This made me change the way I felt and thought about people.

Anyway, back to Donald Trump.

I have a fantasy. I want to become a famous dawnkey. I want to be known by one name: Kaffy. That would be lovely. I would write this book and people would buy it and it would do well and I would become famous and be known as Kaffy, the DawnKey who loves everybuddy!! And I would tell people about my story and how I went from a donkey to a DawnKey with universal love for all.

Trump would hear about me, and that I am a liberal dawnkey. This would amuse him. He would want to know if he, too, is loved by the dawnkey who CLAIMS! to love everybuddy! And he would arrange to meet me, and I can imagine them wanting to do photos and all that stuff and how they'd be searching me and other weird stuff.

But all I'd have is love to offer.

And I would meet him and he would feel a strange charm and trust in this silly, loving woman. And I would tell him I'd like to advise him spiritually, and he, mesmerized, agrees, and we hug and everything is magical and nice.

And the world is stunned.

And everybuddy wants to see the Dawnkey Who Loves Everybuddy!

And God and the universe or whatever you call it will give me the extra special majickal oomph that I need.

I understand that Moses
stuttered.

I give you, reader, the benefit of
the doubt and trust you
understand what I just meant as
it relates to me.

I want to be Kaffy, the Magickal
Love Dawnkey.

I tell you otherwhere in this book
about my feelings about my past
life. I believe I was stressed
sitting here at this window typing
away because I would imagine
the cops or...somebody...coming
for me. I was terrified of that
doorbell, the banging on the door.
I really honestly believe I was
hiding too, from the Nazis, and
was taken somewhere horrible.

When my psychic friend confirmed that I had indeed been in that kind of life, I felt like a weight was taken off my shoulders. I felt like having the window open.

So I have this delusional fairy tale fantasy about being The Love Dawnkey. And affecting people positively and affecting positive changes and talking to rich people and convincing them to take large portions of their money and do practical, humanitarian things with them.

It is like delusional, bipolar crazy thinking. But I take my medication religiously. No pun intended. Funnily, I realized recently I often say things that can be taken two different ways. I don't do this on purpose. It has caused problems I suspect.

Anyway, this book is the mind of a bipolar, schizo affective Dawnkey having a COVID TRUMP DEATH experience.

What has COVID, TRUMP, and DEATH done to me the last 5 years? It has made me into the DawnKey I am today.

So I will begin by dedicating this paper to the following people who have passed:

My father, Jesse Franklin "Frank" Heath

My friends, Janet Ast, Ren Nawee, Amy Burns, Susan Jeswine O'Shea, Susan Himebaugh, Frances Young, Hector Elizalde, Cindy McNash ,

Sally Shoaf, and others. If I have omitted anyone rest assured it is due to my dingbattiness and not their lack of standing in this list.

WEIRDNESS

There was this guy.

This was back around 2008 or so.

I'm going to call him Ooze, because he was slimy like a snail, and to protect his privacy.

I did not know Ooze's name. All I knew was his email address. He was annoying and made my neck hairs stand up. (Not really, but it gives the right ambiance)

So naturally I tried to find out more about him, to no avail. His email, searched on the web, came up with nothing.

Sometimes I get "messages" (in my head.) One day I was sitting at the computer and DING! This name popped in my head. It felt like a message.

At first, I didn't know why I 'got' that name. I didn't know who it was. So, I thought about it for a minute and then it hit me. It was The Ooze!!

Yes, his name came to me out of the clear blue sky and I don't know why. I typed it in with his email address and got a hit. I found a site where he had posted some Ooze and it had his name and email address on it.

What do ya think about THAT?

Essay Compilation: This is Why We Can't Have Nice Things

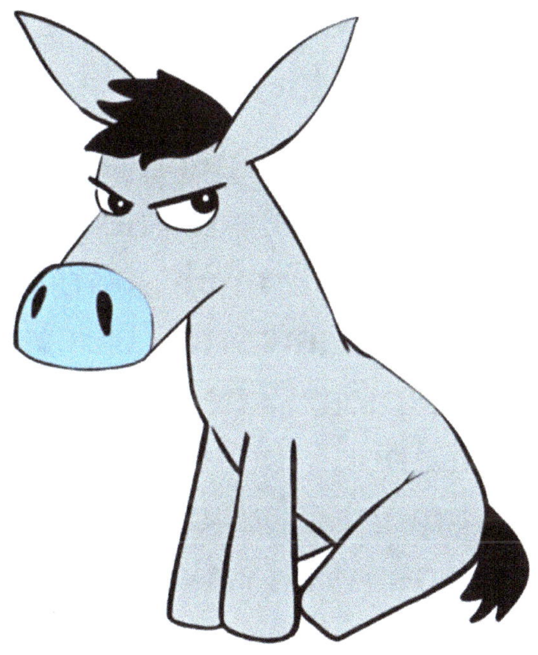

ESSAY #1: THOSE WHO SPILL THE MILK

When I was a teen or something I read the book The Women's Room by Marilyn French (BTW, I recommend it).

Despite the connection of The Women's Room to the feminist movement, French stated in a 1977 interview with The New York Times: "The Women's Room is not about the women's movement... but about women's lives today."[5] (Wikipedia)

There is a part in the book that I was always struck by, amongst others, and it caused an

---

[5] https://en.wikipedia.org/wiki/The_Women%27s_Room

expression to form between my mother and me.

A mother is having issues with her daughter. Her daughter spills the milk and because she feels guilty, acts like a jerk all day. The mother says wearily to herself, "She spills the milk, and I have to pay all day," or something like that.

Mom and I refer to that as spilling the milk.

Some people are like that. They screw up and YOU have to pay. All the doo-damned day.

The human mind is a complex thing it seems. One would think when one screws up the appropriate response is to apologize to those it hurts (if indeed it does). This seems pretty straightforward to me. Tell me if I'm wrong.

But sometimes things go wrong, and pride gets in the way.

Stupid ass pride. It seems a necessary component of the psyche, because good pride is a good thing. Everyone should have good pride ("should" meaning it is beneficial to them) and feel good about themselves and their accomplishments.

Maybe people who do this aren't in touch with themselves... could be some of them don't even know it's bothering them...they are just being a jackass and don't even know why.

sigh I'm not a psychiatrist. I don't know all the answers. I can't figure out what to tell people so they can deal with this problem. All I can do is love people. And maybe that's enough.

What have your experiences been like with this phenomenon, the Milk Spiller? What do you tell someone who is angry because THEY screwed up?

Well, *I* think it's a good idea to sympathize with them.

Yes, even though they are being a pill, bite the bullet and sympathize. Be as warm and understanding and listen-y as possible.

This suggestion may outrage you because it blames the victim or

makes the victim responsible etc.
I tend to use what works...

However, you may find this:
when all the warmth and
understanding has been
transferred to the crabbyass, they
begin processing it and realize the
error of their ways. Because of
your understandingness, they
may scrutinize themselves and
then apologize and mean it.

This is not to say that ANY of this
is your truth. This is my truth.

Let's not get started on the use of
personal truth. That's for another
time.

This has been brought to you by a
group of a series of essays, the
compilation of which I think I will

call, "This Is Why We Can't Have Nice Things!"

BTW, I noticed I use a lot of words to soften what I have to say, because I anticipate being argued with or attacked. It seems like no matter how much I try not to, something slips in that I casually say without thinking. So, I hope I haven't done that.

Happy hump day. Go out there and love someone. Even if they DO spill the milk.

ESSAY #2: SOMEBODY ALWAYS GETS BUTTHURT

Ya know?

No matter what I say, no matter what I do, SOMEbuddy is going to misunderstand or be offended by something I say.

Now, I'm not out there spewing angry stuff and wanting to fight. I try, ♪ oh my God do I try ♪ not to hurt or aggravate or alienate people. But it seems like no matter how careful I am, someone nitpicks or gets upset or misunderstands or something. Or maybe even misses the whole damned point. (I do *SO* have points!)

I will digress a second: I HATE being misunderstood!

"I'm just a soul whose intentions are good, oh Lord please don't let me be misunderstood."

I had a realization just now. Maybe people expect more from me because I am more vocal and heard than some other quieter people, and because I'm out blabbing my head off to everybuddy, it makes my opinion more heard, and therefore more likely to offend someone because they know everyone is hearing it and may be influenced by it. I can see why I need to express more personal responsibility.

Did that make sense?

Because me, I just want to share. I want you to know what is in my head.

Why?

Well, I think I require intimacy.

I am one of those people who want to be completely honest and forthright. Sharing my feelings, and having you respond and say, "Hey! I feel so and so way!" makes me feel close to you. I like hearing your comments. I love it, actually. I feel close to you. I want to feel close to everybuddy. I am a hog for that, I admit it.

I will give you TMI, if I am allowed. So, I need to be told when I am doing that.

I'm going to share something private with you.

I was a listener on a site for people who needed help. I would try to comfort them.

Someone came along and said he was attracted to...

well, someone he ought not to have been. For sake of their privacy, I won't specify that.

But what I want to share with you is what I did. This really should go under the Boundaries essay. (LOL, essay for lack of a better word)

I told him this person was off limits but that they could love them. They could experience the most wonderful love and intimacy with them without being sexual.

So he listened.

I wove a blanket of love and coziness and wrapped it around him, verbally. That's the best way I have of describing it. It was warm, loving, caring...and platonic.

When I was done verbally showing him love, I asked him, "Now isn't that better than sex?"

(Yes, I know that's reaching.)

But! He responded with vigor, YES!! It was wonderful and it was the best thing ever! We then talked more about it and how great it felt. He was able to go on from there and take that with him, and he never tried to push my boundary I set up. (I'd immediately set a boundary because I didn't want to be flirted with. I wasn't there in that capacity.) He didn't try to get me to talk about sex!! I was thrilled and inspired that I had this experience.

I digressed to tell you that so you could understand how I feel about intimacy.

The cost of intimacy is that sometimes people get butthurt.

I hope that I never, ever hurt you or hurt your feelers.

And that is all I have to say about the subject.

For now.

Essay #3: What's Wrong With People?

It's so much easier to just love people.

My friend's dad said, and it made such an impression on my father, "Everybody has problems."

It's like the Good Will Hunting scene. Keep saying it to yourself until it sticks in your head and the lightbulb comes on: Everybody has problems.

I used to work as a courier. Sometimes someone would ask me for directions in the building I worked out of. I would draw a map or show them a map and show them exactly how to go.

INVARIABLY someone would show up and say no no no, don't do it like that, let me tell you.

FINALLY, it came to me: people are not always honest. Not everyone knows how to read a map. This had never occurred to me. I assume everyone knows what I know, and more. The guy couldn't come up and say, "Maybe you'd do better with verbal instructions...may I tell you the directions?" Or something like that. And nobody seems to say, "I don't understand maps. Can you tell me a different way?"

So, you have to figure these things out for yourself...why people are doing what they are doing. This is a challenge.

(See, it was okay to push me rudely out of the way, but not to insult the driver's ego by suggesting he may not be able to read a map.)

People hide things.

They have challenges as children, like dyslexia, e.g. Someone may have treated them unfairly because of it. They may be even ashamed. They grow up learning to hide it, because it's like a disability that keeps them from keeping up with the rat race, so to speak.

Some people never learned to read. I knew such a man. He was born poor, married poor, had ten kids, and left behind real estate and money to his wife when he died. He worked his butt off. He

drove all the way to Florida. I
never noticed any problem. He
couldn't read road signs but he
knew what things looked like. His
wife helped him.

He had to make do with what he
had. He didn't go around telling
people he couldn't read. He didn't
go around telling people about
his problems.

I remember when we owned the
medical equipment business. I
was working one day in the office
and an elderly man came in.
There was some paperwork he
needed to read. I immediately
thought of the aforementioned
man, and without thinking I
asked trying-to-be-helpfully if he
would like me to read it to him.

He became instantly furious and said he could read!

And I looked at him and thought, "My papaw can't read. Who do you think you are, acting like that's a disgrace?" It angered me. But instead, I apologized, kissed butt, and was mortified, too, that I had hurt his feelings. It's not that I thought he couldn't read. It's that I know when you hit middle age your eyes start going, it seems. And when you're elderly, well...lots of patients would ask me to read stuff to them.

But anyway, yeah. People have problems. And they may hide them.

That's why I recommend the Dawnkey Method of Loving Everybuddy.

Because you don't know why they may be doing what they are doing. You don't know their fears, their anxieties, their challenges, all these kinds of things and more, that make them up.

I was about to wrap this up, and I remembered someone.

Years ago, when I was taking care of a lady, her husband was a thorn in my side, and heartache.

He did not seem to like me. He certainly did not like when I coughed (I smoked. Outside. Rarely.) He was gripey and mean spirited and complainy. Once he complained because I made their meals look too nice. What else did I have to do? I didn't have enough work to do.

The wash was always done by another shift before I could do it. I would have loved to have done the wash as it would have been something to do. He comes to me and says "I see others washing the clothes, how come you don't?"

One time his daughter made a roast and overcooked it. He complained BITTERLY. To me, of course. He thought I had cooked it. His daughter spoke up and told him it had been she. He immediately perked up and said, "OH, it's WONDERFUL!!"

I won't go on and on. He was just a jerk.

But I found out why. He had been responsible for the death of his child.

He never got over it.

You just don't know WHY. Don't know all the reasons.

So, you have to give people the benefit of the doubt.

Employee behind the desk in the surgery waiting room: I'm sitting and she calls my name and mentions insurance. I panic. For reasons. She sees my panic.

She informs me that I have blown her hair back. She jumps me verbally.

I stared at her, horrified, and then it hit me. "Are you having a bad day?" I asked kindly.

She didn't say another word. She immediately went into Adulting mode. She immediately checked herself and was extra kind and friendly to everyone who came in after that.

All it took was that one kind sentence and she knew I was sympathetic.

I would much rather have that outcome, than a fight on my hands. Who would win? Who cares? It would be miserable and gut wrenching. Why not be peaceful and loving and affect a positive change?

Essay #4: Can We Have a Utopia? No!!

Why not, you ask?

Because there are asshats out there, and THEY DON'T WANT ONE.

That's right.

Our beautiful utopia, that we could afford if things were done more humanely, is probably not going to happen any time soon, because jerks.

I want it all, dammit. I'm going to try to remember to attach a copy of Maslow's Hierarchy of Needs[6].

---

[6] Hierarchy of needs as presented by Hannah Shannon can be found after Essay #5.

I want all these needs met. For everybuddy. So that everybuddy can work on self-actualization, which is what we are here for, in my opinion.

There is no reason why we can't have health care for all, and proper care for those who need it. There is no reason why all the mentally ill people who got turned out into the street because Reagan closed down the mental hospitals in CA should have to live homeless and uncared for. No reason why people should have to go hungry.

Why can't we have nice things? Well, for one reason, because people steal.

It would be so great to have grocery stores everywhere that

have free food in them. For the poor. Not for people who think, "haha! I can have free stuff! So, I will! Because I can!" but for the poor.

We can't have it, because Jerks. It would be great if people didn't lie and cheat, too. It would be nice if these stores were on the honor system and people who were not going hungry would stay away. But they won't. "It's my right!" "It's legal!" "Where do you draw the line?" blah de blah de blah.

I remember being told by my first in-laws that I should go get the government cheese that was being given out.

I said, "I don't need it and feel bad about taking it."

"Oh, go on and take it! That's what it's for!"

NO, IT'S NOT. It's not an effing free for all! I didn't need that gift, and didn't want to take what I didn't need, possibly resulting in taking it from some poor old family that showed up too late.

Why do people have to think like this?

Why do people camp outside Walmart on Black Friday?? And then hurt each other.

For things.

THINGS!

"People are loving things and using people."

I don't mind capitalism. Not per se. I think it can live in harmony with socialism. But $#@! Why do people have to be so greedy and thoughtless?

There is a percentage of us that does not want utopia. They want to keep making money hand over fist, buckets full, more than they can ever spend, and don't care what the hell happens as long as they get their effing money. And anyone who doesn't have their "Tool Kit," as I call it, and is able to succeed financially, well, screw them. As long as they keep gobbling up resources.

Gobble, gobble, gobble.

Now it's back to Dawnkiness. You know what I think? They're looking for love.

Oh, they don't realize it, likely. Love can get perverted. I don't *necessarily* mean sexually.

Maybe 45 was not reared properly. Perhaps he didn't get the love that he needed.

Maybe that's his problem.

Which makes me think of Elon Musk. What ails him? Well, it just now (I'm ashamed to say) occurred to me to wonder this. So I went and found this:

"Bullied as a Child

Musk attended the private, English-speaking Waterkloof House Preparatory School—he started a year early—and later graduated from Pretoria Boys High School. 9 The years were

258

lonely and brutal, from his descriptions."[7]

I don't need to post his history to make my point.

Aw, God, why can't we all just get along?

Everybody's got problems.

This is why we can't have nice things.

____

[7] https://tinyurl.com/Investopedia-Elon-Musk

ESSAY #5: "LIARS AND THIEVES AND PSYCHOPATHS, OH MY!"

I used to say I hate liars. Or thieves. Psychopaths are so bad that you'd just assume it.

You'd be wrong.

I'm not even sure if I ever hated anybody, and as far as I *know* I've never known any psychopaths.

Sometimes I see it said that sociopaths and psychopaths are the same thing.

Website Quote:

"The common features of a psychopath and sociopath lie in their shared diagnosis: antisocial personality disorder. The DSM-5 defines antisocial personality as someone having three or more of the following traits:

Regularly breaks or flouts the law

Constantly lies and deceives others

Is impulsive and doesn't plan ahead

Can be prone to fighting and aggressiveness

Has little regard for the safety of others

Irresponsible, can't meet financial obligations

Doesn't feel remorse or guilt"[8]

---

[8] https://mhanational.org/conditions/personality-disorder

I'm impulsive and don't plan ahead.

I'm irresponsible and can't meet financial obligations

That's 2/3 of the necessary diagnostic criteria.

#3: remorse and guilt.

Now there's a bit of a sticky wicket.

I think if I am honest with myself and you, I will admit that I have a high opinion of myself and don't tend to feel remorseful or guilty as much as I seem.

Let's cut to the chase: it sounds like I'm trying to say I have antisocial personality. But in my Cancerian side-ways-moving way, I am trying to say the opposite.

Y'all know me pretty well. Some of you probably better than I know myself. Because I'm an open book. All you have to do is ask. I think you guys know I'm not a sociopath or psychopath.

It makes one wonder though... If I came so close to the cusp, and I'm such a nice little dawnkey, what of others? What if one of my friends who shares my 1 and 2 traits, and throws in the aggressiveness trait? That's 3. That's all that's required.

So, take me, make me mad a lot, and I will have antisocial personality?

OK, I'm obviously not a psychology doctor or a logic student. But it just seems to me that a large percentage of the population may have 3 of those traits. Does it seem like it to you?

So, what makes a sociopath or a psychopath? It sounds to me like a lot of people fit the bill.

Back to my hating/not hating. I've been murderously angry before. But when I give it serious thought, it doesn't seem like I'm much of a hater.

That's why I have to admit I don't hate these people.

<have you ever noticed I process while I write? Carry on>

I'll go a step further and say I don't hate anybody. Not even people who hurt me. Not horrible, sickening people. Nobody. I hate nobody.

I even try to love them. The worst of the worst, the ones we'd want to see snuffed. I say try because I don't want to be attacked for saying I love evil people.

I spent 10-15 years working on my psyche, my soul, etc. In that time miraculous things happened. And I trained myself. I decided what/who I wanted to be, and I faked it 'til I made it. I was a donkey who became a DawnKey. And I believe what I say.

Why do people do evil?

Probably lots of reasons. I won't try to list them all. Maybe some people are born with brains that are malformed or malfunctioning. Maybe others experience brain injuries from falls and other assorted things that happen.

Maybe some people learn it. But things can be unlearned, oh boy can they.

I know someone who fit almost all those categories. They aren't like that anymore. They grew and learned.

They grew and learned. Life was hard for them, but they improved and are a good-hearted soul.

What does that say for society?

Some people are abused horribly, psychologically, verbally, physically, all kinds of ways are possible. Maybe they also get a brain injury.

Nothing happens to their moral system.

Another person has the same thing happen to them, and goes out and kills a bunch of people.

Is it their moral system, though? Or is it something biological, physiological? Is it their soul? Their spirit? What is hurt? What is hurting them? What did hurt them?

I have all these questions and more.

Does their Life's Tool Kit help or neglect them? (I like to call our resources our tool kit. Resources come in all forms.)

Hear the story of Jennings Michael Burch: he wrote *They Cage the Animals at Night.* He was in and out of homes and institutions because his mother was too sick to care for them constantly. The story is painful and beautiful. There is plenty of yuck and some really bright moments.

It's the bright moments we cling to.

A friend recently said it made her day when a stranger greeted them. That's the stuff we remember: kindnesses. And I will remember what she said, because she was more pleased than I expected. And that encourages me to greet others with the same warmth and friendliness and make them feel good...

Jennings had a stuffed dog. They caged the (stuffed) animals at night, so they wouldn't turn up missing. He hid his and made his way out of the institution with him (my heart popdawnks here). He still had him as he wrote the story. That little dog got him through trauma. And so did his friends. And the people who did small kindnesses for him. He remembered, and told us. And now I tell you.

These things all matter.

People remember the kind things you do for them. Maybe your child brings home a friend who is starving at home. And you feed that child, every day.

That will warm that child's heart when he is in distress. He will cling to The Kindnesses.

Gosh, it's so. Damned. Important. To be kind. Go out of your way.

Make it awesome. Be somebuddy's memory!! Their memory of YOU might be the tipping point that makes them do the right thing.

Some people may be just born bad. Like a monster. I don't know why that happens. Something genetic? I don't know much about these things; I just find them compelling.

Does that person deserve to be brutalized?

If he was born that way?

Does a snake deserve to die because it swallows adorable creatures? It was born that way.

So, what do you do with the "monsters" as people call them.

Are they people with no soul? Is that even possible?

Too many concepts here to process all at once.

I want to go back to the kindness issue.

I think if you make it your business to be kind to people on a regular basis, you'll become addicted to it and want more. And as time goes by, you'll feel more and more love.

That's what I wish for you.

Maslow's Hierarchy of Needs

Self-Actualization

I have realized my full moral and creative potential. I am accepted, and have accepted myself. I live life with purpose and meaning.

Esteem

I am confident. I am unique. I respect myself, and others respect me. I have, and will continue to, achieve my goals.

Love and Belonging

I am loved. I give love. I have deep connections with my friends and family. I share intimacy with those I love.

Safety

I am healthy. I am safe. I am secure, physically and financially. I have support from my family, friends, and society.

Physiological

I am fed. I am hydrated. I have shelter over my head and clothes on my body. I can breathe. I can sleep.

UFO Weirdness

I never understood latitude and longitude before, and certainly would not have known where 45 85 or 90 was. I also did not know about Sturgeon Bay and that this area was a UFO capital, until I had this weird dream.

I dreamed I was flying and using something like my pillow...I was resting up in some trees...it was getting gooshy though, coming apart inside, and I had to come down.

I got the message that I would be coming down a little too quickly, down past Indiana, going north, landing in Michigan.

Then I got this number: 45 90.

I landed oddly softly, and there was an old salty guy there, like a sea captain or ex-navy or AirForce or something. He told me disturbing things, and said he could tell me things that would really shock me.

When I woke up and went to the bathroom I remembered the number. SO, I went and looked it up. I thought, wouldn't it be funny if it WERE around Indiana and Michigan? Of course, you know where it is. Right around Sturgeon Bay. I was more stunned when I Googled the area and found that it is a UFO capital area.

So that is my weird tale.

Our Roommate

She's a member of the family, so I won't say her name.

She's been getting... bold lately.

When I try to use the bathroom, she appears and demands things. I'm sitting there, vulnerable, and every. single. time. she comes and takes advantage.

She's jealous of Rick and me, I just know it.

I've found her hair all over his pillow.

She has...this is so shameful...BITTEN me.

Yes!

Rick and I have been snuggling and of course, here she comes.

Hops in Rick's lap!!

Rubs all over him!!!

And then, the coup de état? She reaches over and BITES me!

I've heard of water therapy in these cases. A spray bottle of water to discourage her. But I just can't do it...

She's been getting bold. She's known for years certain things are off limits, like the dining room table and the end tables, e.g.

Found her hair ALL OVER the top of the dining room table! Now WTH is going on there?

And the other day, she got so excited when I was stroking her lovely, soft hair that she jumped up on the end table! Of course, I immediately fussed at her because she knew better, and she jumped down.

I'm so tired of cleaning up after her in the bathroom, but that's part of the agreement, the conditions of her living with us, so it is what it is.

She never complains about the food or drinks I give her. I'm always serving her the same thing, and she never turns up her nose or looks like she doesn't like it. It's so sweet. And she never, ever makes a mess. She's rather quite elegant.

One odd thing she does is walk in front of me every time I try to go into the kitchen. She goes very slowly, switching back and forth.

She reminds me of this girl who used to harass me at school. I keep telling her she's going to trip me and I'm going to fall and break my butt.

She's short. She is a little sensitive about it, I suspect. I never make fun of her about it.

She doesn't mind when I sing. I sing terribly, lol. But I love to sing so much! So, I make up lyrics to popular tunes.

Nowadays we try to include her in our snuggling. She hops up and sits on one of our laps and we scritch her hairy back with our fingers and she's in heaven.

I won't say her name... but her nickname is Kitty.

ROMEOW

This is a poem I wrote for my lovely friend Colleen back at ICHC, using lol speak. (The language we made up on ICHC) Her name there was Romeow, which was the name of her beautiful white floofy cat. For Colleen's birthday I wanted to do something special but all I had was my silly little donkey heart, and so I expressed my feelings...in a primitive way so it would be accepted. Does that make any sense?

Romeow

It r Romeow's Birfday.

*the donkee is all alone and tinks

she cannutt bee herd*

Is quiet, and

Her is thinkeeng abowt her
Romeow.

Shhhh…u kin heer hurr fots if u
lissen

wiff ur hart:

"Oh, Romeow

u is a star

u shine so brite, so brite

u is a lite.

And insite.

U sends mee wurds

u fink r nuffin speshull

an i sits an stares at dem

an dey vibrates wiff a magnetism

(sumtimes like wen i reeds mah
Good Book

its kind ub like dat)

an u say

oh, donkey wut a bootifull thing

an turn it into a lettur

dat i wunt to frame

u mek mee feel 5 an wunt to
SING

U fly froo teh sky

wiff no feer

and I

has a hart full ub lub

an eyes full ub teers as I sings

u gibs ME wings!

and, oh! U meks such bootifull
fings

why,

i fink i wud find dem at teh fantsy
place

or sumplace furr ellebentee
thousand dollars

butt dem is priceless.

an Romeow teh cat

Rest him soul

looks down an crais

wiff joy dat hee gotted too bee
yur bebbeh

How prowd hee muss bee

Hee shows all him frens

an points wiff floofeh arm

Look, dat MAH hyoomun

an has a prowd

an dey nod sollumlee

wiff big eyes

sumtams i marvels how life can
bee so byootifull,

an den u comes along and turns
up teh shine.

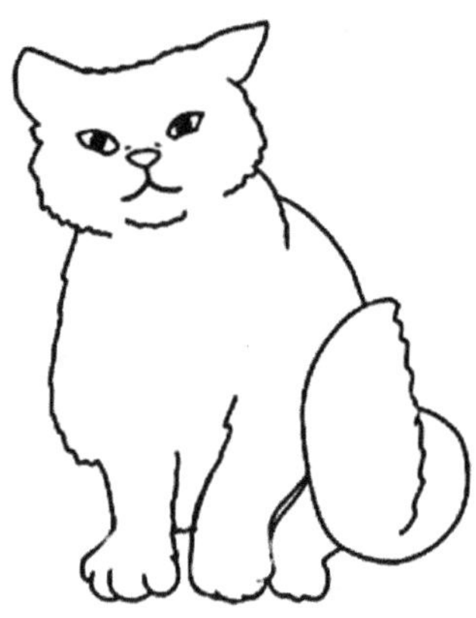

Dad and I

Hi everybuddy. I just spent the last hour writing this. It poured from me. It is about my father, and a lot about me, too. And how we came to be good friends in the end. It is terrifically long, and I don't expect anyone to read it, but it feels like something I need to post. For myself. It's very, very personal. So, you've been warned. Bless you if you read the whole thing.

My father and I had always had a relationship that was difficult for me. He was naturally authoritarian, and I was naturally mousy in response.

Something magical happened, though, when he became permanently bedfast and I began visiting him regularly for several hours at a time. He began to really KNOW me; know the person I had become. And I began to feel adored, a novel feeling in this relationship. We became real and true friends.

We had never really understood each other. But as we shared things that were emotionally important to us, I was able to learn new things about him, and the things I couldn't understand, I was able to just set aside without a worry. I came to accept that he had ways that we could not understand but that wasn't his fault and to just love him for what he was. (Things like this come obvious to those with common sense, but I never really had much.)

And what a man he was. He wasn't like Everybody Else. He was different. He was special. Actually, both my parents fit that description. They are both two special people. I always felt that they stood out in their own unique ways. They are excellent people.

So, striving for perfection it seems in retrospect, these very human people did their utmost to bring me up and in as wonderful an atmosphere as possible. What went wrong?

I have come to the conclusion that, early in life, I decided to model after my father. This didn't always serve me well, and conflicted with the part of me that was like my mom, and the result? Quirky, sarcastic, reserved, and I always felt like I was what they now call "cringey." An oddball.

I never felt comfortable in my own skin until lately. I felt like a little weirdo. Someone with the very different traits of Brenda, my mom, and Frank, my dad. And I was trying to be someone I wasn't.

Ironically, I chose the Donkey as an internet avatar and began making friends while schmoozing about in a donkeyish sort of fashion, while occasionally throwing in a story or two or something lovely or touching, and after a while made some friends who genuinely cared and were caring people. And together, we all created an atmosphere on a lolcat site that was loving and playful and (mostly) kind while being fun and funny. I have met some of these people. They are good people.

This was a huge process for me. I was beginning about a 10-15 year (?) process of changing into the me of me.

In the meantime, I had issues. Alcoholism was one. And feeling like a child and a failure in my parents' house. And worshipping them both and not wanting to fail them, or ever, ever tell them no. And overeating. And not having that much of the physicality to do the kinds of help they needed from me.

So, one night, I was trying to help dad with the computer. We were both drunk. He misunderstood me and then accused me of calling him a liar, if I remember correctly. The very idea that I would call my Father a liar!!! We were soon enmeshed in a furious argument, something that NEVER happens. Soon it became apparent to me that he felt scornful toward me, like I was an animal, and I reminded him I was his daughter. He responded hatefully. In another few words, I was in my room, in a fury, and I sought a tool to cut myself as badly as I could manage.

Fortunately, I ended up in the hospital, and in a psych ward. It was an incredible experience. They diagnosed me as I suspected: bipolar. When I arrived, I was on a gurney, and I couldn't stop crying. I just lay there, not caring, on the thing, and crying and crying. I was so incredibly depressed. Patients gathered around. Someone helped me down to sit in a chair. I was so huge. I couldn't fit. And she said, "Oh, you're too tall," and I think this act of kindness made me cry again.

I was also mildly delusional. Some point I shifted. And I became sort of grandiose feeling. And I had no shortage of patients knocking on my door and

wanting me to come out and play.
I felt like the Donkey, and some
students came and wanted to
know if they could interview
some of us patients. And I agreed.
I told a glorious tale of High
Donkiness. I came alive in there
and made friends and felt like I
understood people, people who
were people, not freaks, and just
had problems, like everyone else.
Everyone has problems.

And I did good things for people,
lots of good things, and some
were small and others more
profound.

And I was finally medicated.

Thus began a shift in my father's
and my relationship. Suddenly he
was more doting. More patient.

And, to my surprise, more respecting.

Another thing was happening: I had a history of poor romantic choices and baggage to go with it. I finally decided I had had it when a guy who was clearly my boyfriend informed me he was NOT. This is when the candy shop got closed down. For ten years. No dating. And as I was growing into a DawnKey, I was learning and striving toward appreciating someone kind. And good. And patient. And affectionate—enough affectionate and lovingness to blot out all the old needy wanty clingy/withdrawing craziness.

And I found the right person. Another person, like me, who

identifies as broken. And together we make perfect. Four years, still no arguing. No fights. Just respectful disagreements.

The last few years have been eye opening spiritually, while being traumatizing, shocking, surprising, depressing, and other nasties. At some point I became almost obsessively spiritually critical, constantly thinking of methods of improvement. And in many ways, I have grown, exceedingly.

This is what my father came to understand. And he came to see me, well, sort of like in the eyes of those who love me. Or something like that?

I don't just post boring inspirational memes and cat pics

all the time. I do good stuff when I can. I promise. I'm a horn tooter from way back, but not this time.

And dad finally came to understand this. His face would light up about it. He never knew about my online life before he was bedfast. He just wasn't interested. And when he was bedfast, he finally got to know me for the true me, and not someone trying to be someone I'm not.

Because, despite the fact that I "act like" a donkey sometimes, I am 100% for realz. I am coming to you from the heart, and honest as you're going to find. I am the product of Frank and Brenda Heath, my own special entity, and I am full of light and love, just

like my mother, and just like dad
is, now, eternally.

To Sean, With Love

Dear Sean,

I'm writing this to let the world know that I was a mess of a mother.

Yet, you flourished as soon as you got out of our clutches. You were like a bloom all trapped and burst out when you were free.

You know I was irresponsible to the end: when I promised God I would no longer drink, I was still being irresponsible. I did not want to have to be responsible and abstain. So, I made a promise that I knew I hadn't the guts to break.

You know all my reasons. You know how I feel. But the

WORLD...you deserve for the world to know. How I neglected you. How I was ugly to you. How I let you cry. How I scared you, because I wanted so badly to share everything with you. I treated you like an adult when you were a child, and that was wrong.

When you were little, I showed you medical pictures you were too young to see. I wanted you to be unusually intelligent so badly.

I tried to teach you organs and things of the human body, when you were just tiny.

I over shared with you.

I sat on that @#$! Computer looking for love, while you ached to have a mom.

I was way too stupid to realize I was only looking for what I already had, and I was ignoring it.

I think I just hit the nail on the head.

I'm so proud to know you, yet so humbled.

I love you,

Mom

Nap and I

Meet my best friend since 3rd grade, Nancy Price. I used to call her Nap.

She is amazing.

She is like me, and not.

She is complex.

I was a twerpy kid. I am not sure what she saw in me. I seem to remember coming down to the creek one day and there she was, doing her Nancy Thing, fishing, catching crawdads, etc. I remember the early days and hanging out with her...I remember her catching a fish one time and we couldn't get it off the hook. It was awful. She told me to look away and she took care of the situation. I've always remembered that. I took it to mean that she was more mature than I, and I was grateful for her grit.

We spent many summers at that creek. It was heaven.

 I was given to silliness and games, sometimes when it wasn't appropriate.

I remember a game I liked to play with her I called Clue. (Totally stealing from the board game.) I would write up a series of clues with puzzles of a sort in them. Then Nancy would go on the search for whatever was at the end. She was always so willing to hang around while I did things.

Nancy would hang around when I did stupid stuff, but didn't join in. I was called a fool more than once. Once I was called a fool when I decided to wrap a Christmas bulb in wire and try to plug it in.

It snapped and popped.

I'm lucky that's all it did.

Sometimes I think she was with me when I would mix things in my chemistry set and then run.

I'm still laughing at her calling me a fool. I was SUCH a fool.

I was not perceptive.

My parents liked to remind me that my cousin Donna was more perceptive than I. I would hear this several times. I wasn't quite sure what to do with the information.

One time, for my birthday, they got me luggage. I think it was my 14th. Anyway, they just put it in the garage. They knew I would never notice it.

Nancy was perceptive. She could lay in the grass and stare at a bug forever. It was fascinating to be with her. Nancy knew stuff about all kinds of things.

She knew about science and told me interesting things. I admired her. My parents admired her. So much so that when her mother died, she came and lived with us down in southern Indiana.

More on that later.

I remember her showing me the book The Painted Bird. I was appalled. It has always stuck in my mind. I marveled at this child who was so dignified, so intelligent, so well read. She knew about things that blew my mind.

I remember her telling me about the OOBE.

I was transfixed with fascination.

OOBE, she explained, was an Out of Body Experience.

I wanted to have an OOBE. I desperately tried, to no avail. I wouldn't be surprised if she were already having them. She was very spiritual. (BTW, I still haven't had one.)

It was just so wonderful to be around her.

I remember with pleasure the scenes of Nancy and me seeing each other on the bicycle path and hurrying towards each other with glee, Nancy's luxurious long blond/brown hair braid flopping against her as she ran towards me.

Sometimes, later, when her mom got to trust me a little, I was allowed in the garage to play. We had great times in there, I remember. Nancy had a little book called, "Isn't It Shocking" or "Shocking Tales" or something. I remember looking at it with great interest. She watched patiently. I opened it and ZAP! It's funny the things you remember and laugh about.

I also remember learning about artistic plagiarism. I'm imagining it was around third grade when I saw a painting her artist brother had done and wanted to try to emulate it. I copied it and showed it to Nancy. Her eyes got big with the I'M FREAKED OUT look. I learned that day that such behavior was not appropriate.

Nancy and I were not fighters. Later as teens we grouched at each other a little, but we never got into physical altercations.

Except.

One time we were playing Mastermind, I think... anyway we were getting silly and either over or under stimulated and got goofy and I made a movement to act like I was going to smack her, as a joke, and I actually did it accidentally.

It was horrible.

I felt like the biggest piece of crap in the universe. I ended up leaving. We didn't see each other for what felt like weeks.

Then one day, here she came, down the bicycle path! She was wearing an orange shirt, and I made a crack about it. How did I have the gall to do such a thing? But she accepted me back and we were friends again.

I loved that orange shirt.

When Nancy was around 14, her mother died. It was awful. Her mother was a beautiful, funny, and interesting person. I liked her so much. I only got to see her a couple or so times, but it was pleasant. I remember wearing size 12 cutoff jeans, and feeling huge in them, and she was complimentary. That made me feel so good.

When Nancy's mother passed, we moved from Indianapolis to Orleans, Indiana. It was horrible, leaving Nancy. Soon afterward, maybe within a year, her father allowed her to come and stay with us, and she did, for the next 3 or so years.

It. Was. Hell.

And I was the demon.

I was too stupid and blind and naive and young to realize what Nancy was going through psychologically. I worried her to death, almost.

It was a long three years, and I am sure it was traumatic at times for her.

In my early 20s, my dad's mother, Grandma Camp, pressured me into not being friends with Nancy. I won't go into the horrid details, but it was sad. I can't believe I did that.

We were separated for many years because of that. But she was still a sister to me, in my heart, the whole time.

In 1997 we moved to San Francisco and I became a voracious internet user. She found me online, and we were thrilled to be friends again and for the most part, have been. She lives far away, so I don't get to see her anymore, but I miss her horribly. I enjoy being able to converse with her online, though.

She's like a sister and deserves mention in this book about my life. My life would have been totally different without you, Nancy. I love you so much.

Conclusion

I know this book hasn't flowed from beginning to end like an autobiography. But that is how my mind works, and I want you to see how my mind works. I want to share that with you, and I feel that I have.

I have so much more to say, but I am afraid. Afraid that if I spend too much time on this book, it will never be finished. I feel two things:

1. Everything is pouring into my brain, like a deluge. I can't write it fast enough.

2. I will write more books. More and more. I have so much to say.

There is so much I haven't shared with you. But that's okay! I have forever to write.

FOREVER.

There are two things I want to impress upon you, my friend:

1. Life goes on forever.

2. Be kind.

That's what I want you to take from this book. If I have inspired you in any way, please, please tell me. You may write to me at:

KAFLEENBYRAM@GMAIL.COM

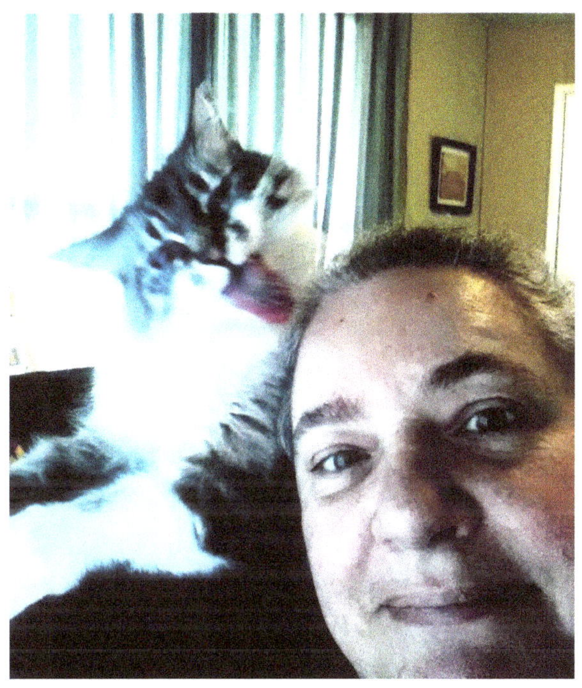

Kathleen Byram lives in Sacramento, CA with her partner Rick and two lively cats. Her loves include scrapbooking, internet surfing, talking, writing, lightworking, and the ocean.